Low-Carbohydrate Mania

The Fantasies, Delusions, and Myths

Richard Harding

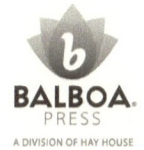

BALBOA.
PRESS
A DIVISION OF HAY HOUSE

Richard Harding
web: www.wisenutritioncoaching.com.au

Balboa Press books may be ordered through booksellers or by contacting:

Balboa Press
A Division of Hay House
1663 Liberty Drive
Bloomington, IN 47403
www.balboapress.com.au
1 (877) 407-4847

Because of the dynamic nature of the Internet, any web addresses or links contained in this book may have changed since publication and may no longer be valid. The views expressed in this work are solely those of the author and do not necessarily reflect the views of the publisher, and the publisher hereby disclaims any responsibility for them.

The author of this book does not dispense medical advice or prescribe the use of any technique as a form of treatment for physical, emotional, or medical problems without the advice of a physician, either directly or indirectly. The intent of the author is only to offer information of a general nature to help you in your quest for emotional and spiritual well-being. In the event you use any of the information in this book for yourself, which is your constitutional right, the author and the publisher assume no responsibility for your actions.

Any people depicted in stock imagery provided by Thinkstock are models, and such images are being used for illustrative purposes only.
Certain stock imagery © Thinkstock.

Print information available on the last page.

ISBN: 978-1-5043-0615-7 (sc)
ISBN: 978-1-5043-0616-4 (e)

Balboa Press rev. date: 06/13/2017

Dedication

This book is dedicated to
Anton Du Plessis

Acknowledgement

Professor Stewart Truswell, Emeritus Professor of Human Nutrition at University of Sydney, has provided advice and encouragement in preparing this book.

Contents

1

Introduction

Numerous popular books, documentaries, websites, and magazine articles passionately advocate different versions of a low-carbohydrate diet. Below are some common "facts" presented by these authorities.

- Serum cholesterol is irrelevant to heart disease. Studies have consistently failed to show evidence that fat, saturated fat, and cholesterol are involved in heart disease.
- The concept that diet and heart disease are linked resulted from corrupt science. Ancel Keys manipulated data to obtain his conclusions regarding fats and heart disease.
- There are no studies to support the claims that saturated fat and cholesterol are involved in heart disease. The idea that saturated fats and cholesterol cause heart disease is the greatest scientific deception of our times.
- Eating saturated fat does not raise your cholesterol.
- Cholesterol in your blood is only harmful if it is oxidized.

- Sugar is the cause of heart disease. Dr John Yudkin is presented as a visionary who linked sugar consumption to heart disease. His views were ignored, or—worse—ridiculed by the establishment.
- Several courageous scientists opposed recommendations for reductions in saturated fat and dietary cholesterol. These heroes were ignored by medical authorities.
- Saturated fats are portrayed is being a great food source because they are stable – they do not become rancid.
- Cholesterol is involved in the healing of heart disease.

These popular ideas are based on myths, fabrications, and distortions of the facts.

Unfortunately, these views have become accepted as the truth. Instead of informing our society about healthy dietary choices, they are causing harm.

Every avoidable illness means a life that is not lived to its full potential.

Every preventable death is somebody's husband, wife, mother, father, brother, sister, or friend whose life is prematurely cut short.

• • • • •

The book is divided into four sections.

The Myths: The second chapter is a review of four popular commentaries regarding diet and heart disease with the third chapter exploring some of the myths that are common in the popular press.

The Basics: Most articles assume that the reader knows about trans-fats, saturated fats, and the foundations of nutritional science. The fourth chapter explains some concepts that are essential in nutrition. A description of the events in a heart attack is explained.

The Research: This section details some of the research that has helped us to understand health and disease in our society. Chapter five gives a brief overview of some investigators in the early development of cardiovascular research with chapter six examining a number of studies that help form our view regarding nutrition and health.

History of Diets: Chapter seven outlines some popular diets, which have been grouped into four groups: low-carbohydrate diets, standard Western diet, Mediterranean diets and whole-food, plant-based diets. Many popular diets belong in the low-carbohydrate diet group.

2

A Review of Popular Commentaries

BBC Documentary: The Men Who Made Us Fat

At the beginning of the three-part documentary *The Men Who Made Us Fat*, Jacques Peretti informs, "I am going to trace those responsible for a revolution in our eating habits. I'll be looking at how decisions made behind closed doors transformed food into an addiction." A brief shot of Ancel Keys and George McGovern are shown as two of the perpetrators of this exploit.

Robert Lustig is a pediatric endocrinologist at the University of California, San Francisco. He is the author of *Fat Chance: Beating the Odds against Sugar, Processed Food, Obesity, and Disease*.[1] He specializes in childhood obesity and studying the effects of sugar in the diet. He is the director of the UCSF Weight Assessment for Teen and Child Health Program and a member of the Obesity Task Force of the Endocrine Society.

Below are some comments by Lustig from the documentary:

> This man, Ancel Keys, claimed he had the answer to heart disease. His theory had a decisive impact on what we would all eat. But it also had a devastating side effect—creating the conditions for obesity.
>
> Keys's theory was that fat alone caused heart disease. [...]
>
> In 1952, Keys did a sabbatical in England where he saw the epidemic of heart disease himself and correlated it with the enormously poor British diet of fish and chips, etc.—you know what I'm talking about—and decided that saturated fat had to be the culprit. And he actually said that back in the fifties before he did any studies. And he spent the next fifty years attempting to prove himself right.
>
> Keys won the battle. Yudkin was thrown under the bus. And—well, he was discredited by numerous societies basically saying that he did not have the data to make his claims about the importance of sugar.[2]

Much of what a rather chubby Robert Lustig states is false.

Firstly, Keys's research was not the starting point for nutritional and cholesterol research, which had its foundations in the early years of the twentieth century.

Keys's early views on diet were formed in Italy and Spain, not in England. He developed his ideas about diet and heart disease when he was invited to Naples in the early 1950s. His studies showed dramatically lower rates of coronary heart disease in Italy and Spain. He introduced the concept of the Mediterranean diet to America—a diet he described as mainly vegetarian.

Initially, Keys did focus on fats in the diet—not saturated fats—as Lustig states above. Keys conducted many trials and experiments, both before and after he came to his initial conclusions regarding fat.

A number of other researchers, including Jeremiah Stamler, Gerry Shaper, Michael Oliver, and Geoffrey Rose, were of the opinion that "there was no firm evidence linking intake of dietary sugar and CHD."[3]

The claim that "Keys's theory was that fat alone caused heart disease" is false and deceptive. Keys noted in 1980, "Responsible students of the coronary problem long ago abandoned the idea of seeking the cause of the disease, agreeing that several, perhaps many, variables are involved in almost all cases."[4] As the title of this report *(Seven Countries: A Multivariate Analysis of Death and Coronary Heart Disease)* indicates, Keys and his colleagues were examining a number of different variables in relation to heart disease.

• • • • •

Lustig states, "Keys was already pretty famous in America because he was the originator, inventor, of the K-Ration.

The K-ration was a way of getting 12,000 calories in a very small, compact little box." Lustig had overestimated the amount of energy in the K-Ration by three to four times. The K-Ration was an emergency survival ration consisting of non-perishable food designed for a few days' use only. The program claims that the K-Ration contained a lot of sweet food like chocolate, "never for one moment [realising that] it could be harmful." As well as chocolate bars, it contained pemmican biscuits, veal meat, sausage, toilet paper, chewing gum, and cigarettes. The K-Ration was never designed for long-term use.

• • • • •

Lustig's claim that Keys made his assertion regarding the implications of fats in the diet with heart disease without the backing of research is not true.

In 1922, de Langen, working with Javanese men in the East Indies, showed that a diet high in eggs, butter, and meat raised serum cholesterol.

Keys performed studies with his wife, Margaret, in Naples and Rome in 1952.

In 1947, Keys commenced the *Minnesota Business and Professional Men Study* to determine why apparently healthy middle-age men were dying from heart attacks. A number of variables were examined, with serum cholesterol being the most significant variable.

A number of researchers studied the relationship of saturated fat to serum cholesterol during the 1950s. J Groen, LW Kinsell, EH Ahrens, A Keys, JM Beveridge and B Bronte-Stewart replaced saturated fats in the diet with polyunsaturated fats. All other components of the diet remained the same and the total fat content of the diet did not change.

When the unsaturated fats, such as corn or safflower oil, were replaced by the saturated fats of butter, lard, or coconut oil, the serum cholesterol rose. The serum cholesterol fell when the polyunsaturated fats were reintroduced. The experiments were repeated, and whilst there was variability with the amount of change for different individuals, the results were consistent for each individual. The changes occurred rapidly within one or two weeks.

Ahrens's study kept the total fats at 40%, which was the average fat intake of the U.S. at that time.

• • • • •

The conclusion of part one of *The Men Who Made Us Fat* states, whilst showing a picture of Ancel Keys, that "another [Keys] gave the risk of sugar a clean bill of health." Keys disapproved of "the common high level of sucrose in many diets."[5] He advocated a Mediterranean-style diet of traditional Greece, Spain, and southern Italy. This diet was high in unprocessed foods, consisted of "pasta in many forms, leaves sprinkled with olive oil, all kinds of vegetables in season," was "almost vegetarian (or lactovegetarian)," and was "much lower in meat and dairy product" than American diets. At no stage did Keys give sugar a clean bill of health. He did indicate was that sugar was not involved in heart disease.

Catalyst Documentary: Heart of the Matter

The Australian Broadcasting Corporation's *Catalyst* program series produced a two-part program collectively titled *Heart of the Matter*. The programs are titled *Dietary Villains* and *Cholesterol Drug War*. These programs were aired during October 2013.[6]

The presenter and co-producer is Dr Marianne Demasi. The medical experts interviewed include Dr Michael Eades, Dr Jonny Bowden, and Dr Stephen Sinatra. Science and medical writer Gary Taubes was also interviewed.

Eades was born in Springfield, Missouri, and educated in Missouri, Michigan, and California. He received his undergraduate degree in engineering from California State Polytechnic University and received his medical degree from the University of Arkansas. Since 1986, Eades has been in the full-time practice of nutritional and metabolic medicine and weight-loss programs. He is an expert in low-carbohydrate nutrition.[7]

Bowden[8] is a nationally known expert on weight loss, nutrition, and health. He is a board-certified nutritionist with a master's degree in psychology and the author of fourteen books on health, healing, food, and longevity, including three bestsellers: *The 150 Healthiest Foods on Earth*

(2007), *Living Low Carb* (2010), and *The Great Cholesterol Myth* (2012), co-authored with Dr Stephen Sinatra.

Sinatra is a cardiologist with over 35 years of clinical practice, research, and study. His career commenced at Manchester Memorial Hospital in Connecticut and included nine years as chief of cardiology, 18 years as director of medical education, seven years as director of echocardiography, three years as director of cardiac rehabilitation, and one year as director of the weight reducing program. In 1987, Sinatra founded the New England Heart Center. He became an advocate of combining conventional medical treatments for heart disease with complementary nutritional, anti-aging, and psychological therapies.[9]

Gary Taubes, born April 30, 1956, is an American science writer. He is the author of *Nobel Dreams* (1987), *Bad Science: The Short Life and Weird Times of Cold Fusion* (1993), and *Good Calories, Bad Calories* (2007), which is titled *The Diet Delusion* in the UK. Taubes studied applied physics at Harvard, aerospace engineering at Stanford (MS, 1978), and received a master's degree in journalism at Columbia University in 1981. His interests have more recently turned to medicine and nutrition.[10]

Taube's published an article, *What If It's All Been a Big Fat Lie?*, in the New York Times Magazine on 7 July 2002. This article espoused the virtues of the Robert Atkins' low-carbohydrate diet.

• • • • •

Demasi opens the program with the assertion:

> I will follow the road which led us to believe that
> saturated fat and cholesterol causes heart disease
> and reveal why it is being touted as the biggest
> myth in medical history.

The program claims that evidence linking saturated fats, cholesterol, and heart disease is based on "bad science".

The program declares that the idea that saturated fat raises cholesterol arose in the 1950s by Ancel Keys.

Firstly, Keys initially implicated fats, not saturated fats, as stated in the program.

Secondly, the link between cholesterol, fats and heart disease was raised much earlier by a number of investigators. This will be examined in greater detail later.

The program maintains that:

> [Keys] compared the rates of heart disease and
> fat consumption in six countries. It was almost a
> perfect correlation—the more fat people ate, the
> higher the rates of heart disease. Except, there
> was just one problem. Keys withheld data for 16
> other countries. Later, when researchers plotted
> all 22 countries, the correlation wasn't so perfect.

According to Eades, "He more or less cherry-picked countries. You could show just the opposite. You could show that the more saturated fat people ate, the less heart disease they had, if you cherry-picked the right countries."

The graph that Eades refers to originates from Keys's paper *Atherosclerosis: a problem in newer public health.*[11]

Cholesterol skeptics, including *Catalyst*, fail to state where the data for the other sixteen countries originated. It is most likely that the program is referring to the paper *Fat In The Diet and Mortality From Heart Disease*[12] (Yerushalmy and Hilleboe, 1957). This paper used data from 22 countries that were sourced by *World Health Organization* for the years 1951–1953. Clearly this information was not available to Keys as his paper was first presented at a conference at Amsterdam in late 1952. The paper was later "repeated to small audience in New York at Mt Sinai Hospital" in January 1953.[13]

Keys also used data from national food balance data for 1949 supplied by the Food and Agriculture Organization, which published data for 41 countries.

Keys plainly stated in his paper why he chose the countries. He did not select his countries from a single repository of information but used a number of sources.

Even if data from *all* the 22 countries are included, it still shows:

- positive correlations between heart disease and total calories consumed, fat consumption, animal fat consumption, animal protein consumption, and
- negative correlations with heart disease and carbohydrate consumption, vegetable protein consumption, vegetable fat consumption.

Yerushalmy and Hilleboe's paper states, "for all categories of heart disease the association is strongest for animal protein expressed in total calories."

Keys's paper will be reviewed later in the book.

• • • • •

The *Catalyst* program claims that heart disease is really the result of sugar consumption. This hypothesis was given much publicity by John Yudkin, professor of nutrition at London University. Yudkin noticed that sugar consumption increased more than any other food component during the first half of the twentieth century and was closely correlated with the increase in cardiovascular disease.

Yudkin published the book *Pure, White and Deadly: the problem with sugar*[14] in 1972.

Gary Taubes claims that:

> Keys was ridiculing John Yudkin and his theory in papers, and just on the basis of that sort of personality and political struggle, the nutrition community embraced this idea that saturated

fat was the problem, working through dietary cholesterol, and began to think of the idea that sugar could heart disease as akin to quackery, and Yudkin was eventually ridiculed.

Keys was not the only person to publish papers critical of Yudkin's analysis. Jeremiah Stamler, Gerry Shaper, Michael Oliver and Geoffrey Rose were prominent researchers who considered that "there was no firm evidence linking intake of dietary sugar and CHD."[15]

Oliver was a leading British cardiologist, who was also a leading critic during this period of the importance given to blood cholesterol in heart disease. He changed his views by the mid-1990s.

This does not mean that Keys approved of the high level of sugar consumption:

> None of what is said here should be taken to mean approval of the common high level of sucrose in many diets. But there are plenty of good arguments to reduce the flood of dietary sucrose without building a mountain of nonsense about coronary heart disease.[16]

• • • • •

The *Catalyst* program *Heart of the Matter* refers to the *Lyon Diet Heart Study* as evidence that cholesterol is not implicated in heart disease.

The *Lyon Diet Heart Study* is a "randomized, single-blind secondary prevention trial aimed at testing whether a Mediterranean-type diet, compared with a prudent Western-type diet, may reduce recurrence after a first myocardial infarction."

Jonny Bowden claims:

> The point nobody talks about. [...] Both groups had the same cholesterol level except one group just stopped dying. So much for the relationship between cholesterol and the risk of heart disease.

It is incorrect to state that "one group stopped dying". The subjects following the Mediterranean-style diet had a 50% to 70% lower risk of recurrent heart disease. There were 16 cardiac deaths in the control group and 3 in the experimental group. The number of non-fatal cardiac events fell from 17 to 5.

The final report of the *Lyon Diet Heart Study* states, "The data confirm the impressive protective effect of the Mediterranean diet." The report concludes:

> Major traditional risk factors, such as high blood cholesterol and blood pressure, were shown to be independent and joint predictors of recurrence.

> [For] each increase of 1 mmol/L of total cholesterol increased the risk of recurrence by 20% to 30%. Epidemiological studies have consistently shown a positive correlation between plasma cholesterol

levels and the incidence of (and mortality from) CHD in various populations. Thus, our population does not appear to be different from other low-risk populations.[17]

This contradicts the conclusion that *Catalyst* derived from the *Lyon Diet Heart Study*.

• • • • •

Catalyst showed recordings of the U.S. Senate Select Committee on Nutrition hearings, chaired by Senator George McGovern. It showed an unnamed, heroic scientist passionately imploring that the guidelines be deferred— "that's why I have pleaded in my report and will plead again orally here for more research on the problem before we make announcements to the American public."

The scientist was Robert (Bob) Olson, professor of medicine and chairman of biochemistry at St. Louis University and a consultant to the American Egg Board.[18]

As a member of the National Academy of Science, Olson co-authored a report *Toward Healthful Diets* that extolled the virtues of the high-fat, high-meat American diet.[19]

McGovern was born in 1922 in small farming community in the south of South Dakota. His father was a Methodist minister, who served the impoverished and hungry communities of South Dakota during the extreme hardships of the depression of the 1930s.

McGovern served as a bomber pilot in Europe during the Second World War, earning an Air Force medal with three Oak Clusters and the Distinguished Flying Cross. McGovern was a skilled pilot and leader, who managed to landed his badly damaged bomber on several occasions— once with his co-pilot friend dead next to him. He was a senator of South Dakota from 1963 to 1980. He was the first director of the Food for Peace program in 1961 and was involved in the creation of the United Nations' World Food Programme. McGovern was the chairman of the Senate Select Committee on Nutrition and Human Needs from 1968 to 1977.[20]

In 1998, McGovern served a three-year term as United States' ambassador to the United Nations' Agencies for Food and Agriculture during President Clinton's administration. He worked with Bob Dole (U.S. Congressman from Kansas, 1961–1996) to create the McGovern-Dole International Food for Education and Child Nutrition Program in 2000.

In 2000, Clinton presented McGovern with the Presidential Medal of Freedom, the nation's highest civilian honor, in recognition of McGovern's service in the effort to eradicate world hunger.

In October 2001, McGovern was appointed as the UN Global Ambassador on World Hunger and remained in that position until his death in October 2012, at the age of 90.

The first draft of the *McGovern Report* (1977), linking heart disease and food, caused such a tumult that major revisions were required before it was released for publication. In the

Catalyst program, Eades claims that "McGovern himself was from a big wheat-growing state, so it didn't hurt him politically that people moved away from foods of animal origin into breads and pastas."

As well is being a large wheat producing state, South Dakota also produces livestock. Much of the grain produced is used to raise livestock. McGovern believed that he and five other senators from agricultural states lost seats in November 1980, partly as a result of this report.[21] McGovern was not re-elected to office— any office — after the November 1980 senate elections. The notion that McGovern was driven by political motives cannot be substantiated and collapse with a little scrutiny.

• • • • •

The conclusion of the *Catalyst* program was, "exercise and a Mediterranean-style diet is the best way to prevent heart disease."

It was Keys who coined the term Mediterranean diet to describe the traditional diets of Spain, Greece and southern Italy.

Keys and his wife Margaret wrote three books extolling the virtues of the Mediterranean diet: *Eat Well and Stay Well* (1959)[22]; *The Benevolent Bean* (1967)[23]; and *How to eat well and stay well the Mediterranean Way* (1975)[24].

TIME Magazine's Article – Eat Butter

According to Bryan Walsh, in a TIME magazine article *Don't Blame Fat*:[25]

> Keys' work became the foundation for a body of science implicating fat as a major risk factor for heart disease. The Seven Countries Study has been referenced close to 1 million times. [...] But Keys' research had problems from the start. He cherry-picked his data.

If the book has really been "referenced close to a million times", it means that it has been referenced nearly 80 times every day, including weekends, since the book was published in 1980.

Walsh claims that Keys "cherry-picked" his data. It is evident that Walsh has confused Keys's 1953 paper, *Atherosclerosis: a problem in newer public health* with his later study, *Seven Countries: A Multivariate Analysis of Death and Coronary Heart Disease.*

Walsh fails to elaborate on how Keys "cherry-picked" his data. Commencing in 1957, the *Seven Countries Study* studied 12,763 men in sixteen regions in seven countries. Walsh fails to specify what data that was omitted from this study and how was the data "cherry-picked."

Keys collaborated with a number of highly regarded researchers—people who spoke the native language of the areas studied. He lists fifteen collaborators in his *Seven*

Countries: A Multivariate Analysis of Death and Coronary Heart Disease book. According to Henry Blackburn:

> At this time, Keys's matchup with great clinicians completed the picture – such leaders as Paul Dudley White of Boston, Vittorio Puddu of Rome, Noboru Kimura of Japan, John Brock of Capetown, Martti Karvonen of Helsinki, and Christ Aravanis of Athens. All saw beyond the clinic and beyond the individual patient – to the origins of common diseases – in the population and in society.[26]

Paul Dudley White was a highly regarded and renowned cardiologist and is frequently viewed as a leader in preventive cardiology. White was actively involved in the selection of the countries and regions for study.

TIME magazine article contends that Keys manipulated data for his own purposes and at the same time managed to deceive, for decades, his collaborators who actually collected the data.

According to Walsh:

> Keys highlighted the Greek island of Crete, where almost no cheese or meat was eaten and people lived to an old age with clear arteries. But Keys visited Crete in the years following World War II, when the island was still recovering from German occupation and the diet was artificially lean. Even more confusing, Greeks on the

neighboring isle of Corfu ate far less saturated fat than Cretans yet had much higher rates of heart disease.

Corfu and Crete are separated by over 600 km of ocean and dozens of islands—they are not neighboring islands. Surveys for the *Seven Countries Study* were conducted in Greece in 1960, 1965 and 1970. This is not in the years immediately following World War II. It is false to state that the diet was "artificially lean."[27]

Cohort	Meat (g/day)	Fish (g/day)	Eggs (g/day)	Cheese (g/day)	Milk (g/day)
Crete	35	18	25	13	235
Corfu	35	60	5	14	70

Consumption of food items

Significant differences in the Cretan and Corfu diet include egg, fish, alcohol, milk, cereal, and potato consumption, which is ignored in Walsh's article. There is also a difference in smoking habits, which is also ignored.

Walsh claims that people of Corfu ate far less saturated fat than the Cretans. The amount of saturated fat is very similar and low. Below is a comparison of data from Crete and Corfu with ten-year death rates.[28]

Cohort	Sample Size	All Causes Deaths	All Causes Death Rate	CHD Deaths	CHD Death Rate	Fat %	Saturated Fat %
Crete	686	42	656	1	9	39	8
Corfu	529	43	833	8	144	33	7
USA Rail	2571	77	1153	146	574	40	18
East Finland	817	147	1864	78	992	39	22

CHD – Cardiac Heart Disease - Death Rate per 10,000

The amount of saturated fat consumed was very similar. Inhabitants of Crete ate more fat, in the form of olive oil. The number of heart disease deaths for both Crete and Corfu were very low.

The Big Fat Surprise – Nina Teicholz

Nina Teicholz is another popular author who claims dietary recommendations are based on "bad science". Teicholz claims:[29]

> In my research I specifically avoided relying upon summary reports, which tend to pass along received wisdoms and, as we'll see, can unwittingly perpetuate bad science. Instead, I've gone back to read all the original studies myself and in some cases have sought out obscure data that were never intended to be found. This book therefore contains many fresh and often alarming revelations about flaws in the foundational work

of nutrition as well as the surprising ways in which it was both ill-conceived and misinterpreted.

What I found, incredibly, was not only that it was a mistake to restrict fat but also that our fear of the saturated fats in animal foods— butter, eggs, and meat— has never been based in solid science. A bias against these foods developed early on and became entrenched, but the evidence mustered in its support never amounted to a convincing case and has since crumbled away.

• • • • •

It is reasonable to suggest that cholesterol and heart disease research originated with Nikolaj Anitschkow. Nina Teicholz reports the situation in the early part of the twentieth century:

> In 1913, the Russian pathologist Nikolaj Anitschkow reported that he could induce atherosclerotic-type lesions in rabbits by feeding them huge amounts of cholesterol. This experiment became quite famous and was widely replicated on all sorts of animals, including cats, sheep, cattle, and horses, leading to the widespread view that cholesterol in the diet—such as one finds in eggs, red meat, and shellfish—must cause atherosclerosis.

This research did not become famous. According to Daniel Steinberg, "his findings were largely rejected or at least not followed up" for over 30 years.[30]

It was not replicated on cats, as claimed (or rats or dogs), for decades because thyroid function in carnivores converts cholesterol into bile salts and does not raise serum cholesterol levels. Dietary cholesterol does increase serum cholesterol in humans that have comparative low initial serum cholesterol levels. "Normal" serum cholesterol levels are much higher in humans than other species.

Teicholz claims that "the hypothesis that saturated fat causes heart disease was developed in the early 1950s by Ancel Benjamin Keys." This another rewrite of the actual history of cardiovascular research.

In the early 1950s, Keys implicated fats, not saturated fats, as being implicated in heart disease. The role of saturated fats was discovered several years in the future.

Keys was certainly not the first person to link diet and fats to heart disease.

• • • • •

Cornelius de Langen worked as a doctor in the Dutch East Indies from 1916-1922. He linked diet, serum cholesterol and heart disease by comparing diets of native Javanese and Europeans. He also noted low cholesterol content of bile and the rarity of gallstone in Javanese.

de Langen performed possibly the first intervention trial relating to diet and serum cholesterol. Five Javanese men were fed a diet rich in eggs, butter and meat for three months. Their mean serum cholesterol rose 30% from 3.3 mmol/L (128 mg/dL).[31]

Lester Morrison in 1946 also linked diet, cholesterol and heart disease before Keys.

Dr John Gofman, a nuclear physicist, was a leading pioneer researcher in the field of lipoproteins who was familiar with Anitschkow's work. His work showed that serum cholesterol and low-density lipoproteins were both indicators of coronary heart disease risk. This work and other evidence convinced Gofman that blood cholesterol, and the dietary determinants of blood cholesterol, were important in atherosclerosis. His wife, Dr Helen Gofman co-authored a low-fat, low-cholesterol diet book[32] that was published in 1951—prior to Keys's paper. John Gofman wrote the preface for the book.

•••••

Teicholz cites Norman Jolliffe's 1957 study, *The Anti-Coronary Club*, as further evidence of the failure of a low-fat diet to arrest heart disease.

The objective of this study was to "determine that a favorable change in the serum cholesterol level produced and maintained by diet would be associated with a favorable change in morbidity and mortality from coronary heart disease."[33] The *Anti-Coronary Club* existed for 14 years—from 1957 until November 1972. There were 814 active experimental male participants and 420 control participants. The control group was started after 2 years after the commencement of the trial.

According to the authors of the study, the intervention with the "prudent diet" was instrumental in achieving "significant and sustained drop in serum cholesterol levels" and "significantly decreased [the] incidence of coronary heart disease."[34]

However, according to Teicholz:

> But then, a decade into the trial, investigators began to find "somewhat unusual" results: twenty-six members of the diet club had died during the trial, compared to only six men from the controls. Eight members of the club had died of heart attacks, but not one of the controls. In the discussion section of the final report, the authors [...] emphasized the improved risk factors among the men in the diet club but ignored what those risk factors had blatantly failed to predict: their higher death rate.

Teicholz cites a paper[35], published in November 1966, to support her claim. She claims the result regarding the mortality rate "was buried in the study report." The results were not buried and are clearly stated, for all to see, in the report. Other papers relating to the trial were also published in 1966.[36] [37]

It was not a decade into the trial. The trial ended in November 1972—and the referenced paper is not the final report. In 1966, the authors were reporting the results for six years of the experimental group and four years of the control group—the control group having started two years later than the experimental group.

The number of *non-coronary* deaths was 18 for the experimental group and 6 for the control group. According to 1966 papers, "the rates for these [non-coronary] deaths in the 50-59 age group were 689 per 100,000 person-years in the experimental group, and 666 per 100,000 in the control group. The difference between these two rates is slight and not statistically significant." Only two deaths occurred in the younger 40-49 age group.

There were 8 new coronary events, which included deaths, for the experimental group and 12 for the control group. This gave an incidence for the experimental group of 339 per 100,000 person-years compared with 980 for the control group. The control group (the group with no intervention) had new cardiac events at a rate of 290% greater than the active group. Given that there are 420 men in the control group and 814 in the experimental group, the number of deaths and incidents cannot be directly compared.

The 26 members did not die in the experimental group: 26 deaths reported by Teicholz is obtained from adding 18 non-coronary *deaths* to 8 new coronary *events*, which included incidents other than deaths. The 6 deaths reported by Teicholz in the control group related only to non-coronary deaths—the coronary deaths were not included.

A later report, published in 1980, shows the incident rates at the end of the study in 1972. For males aged 40-49, the incidence for new events was 465 per 100,000 in the experimental group compared with 784 per 100,000 in the control group. For males aged 50–59, the incident rates were 1,309 and 2,010 per 100,000 respectively.[38]

Only 19% of the experimental group had *no* risk factors for heart disease compared with 34% for the control group. The three risk factors, associated with heart disease, were: cholesterol 260 mg/dL (6.7 mmol/L) and greater; diastolic high blood pressure 95 mmHg or greater; and obesity. Despite the experimental group having a much higher level of risk factors, their participants had much better outcomes than the control group. The goal was to reduce total fat intake from 40% calories to 33% of calories and reduce saturated fats. Note that these risk factors and goals were very conservative—optimal goals are lower.

• • • • •

Another criticism by Teicholz, printed in the Wall Street Journal, contends:[39]

> Critics have pointed out that Dr Keys violated several basic scientific norms in his [Seven Countries] study. For one, he didn't choose countries randomly but instead selected only those likely to prove his beliefs, including Yugoslavia, Finland and Italy. Excluded were France, land of the famously healthy omelette eater, as well as other countries where people consumed a lot of fat

yet didn't suffer from high rates of heart disease, such as Switzerland, Sweden and West Germany.

Teicholz is another popular author who contends that Keys selected the countries to confirm his existing beliefs in isolation from others.

Random clinical trials are a useful tool to determine the effectiveness of an intervention such as the prescription of a drug, the effectiveness of a procedure, or the intake of a vitamin. Participants are randomly assigned to a control (no intervention) group or to an experimental (intervention) group. A comparison of the outcomes between the two groups can then be evaluated.

It is difficult to determine how an effective long term observation trial could be designed where the countries are selected randomly. The first two countries selected for the *Seven Countries Study* were Finland and Japan. They were selected because, at the time, they were the countries with the highest and lowest mortality rates from heart disease. North Karelia in Finland was selected because it had the highest mortality rate in Finland. North Karelia is an inland region in East Finland that borders Russia. A contrasting region was chosen on the coast in south-west Finland. The two Japanese regions were located on the southern island of Kyushu. Tanushimaru is a rural farming community and Ushibuka is a contrasting costal village with a high fish intake.

The *Seven Countries Study* did not compare countries. It compared sixteen contrasting regions in seven countries. If countries (or regions) were chosen randomly, it is possible to obtain two similar, adjacent regions that would provide a limited amount of useful data. Other factors that were considered included the associations with local speaking collaborators and availability of funding. Randomly selecting the countries is not a useful or appropriate methodology for such a study.

In the introduction of *Seven Countries* (1980) publication and *Coronary heart disease in seven countries (1970) I. The Study Program and Objectives*, Keys documents in great detail how the sixteen contrasting regions in the seven countries were selected. The eligible participants in the study were all men of the ages 40–59. An average of 95.9% of all eligible men participated in the study—except for the cohorts in the Netherlands and the U.S.

Netherlands was included, despite the anticipation that it would uncover results contrary to their expectations:

> Netherlands was later included because government agencies in that country offered personnel and financial help and because the official statistics of the Netherlands in the mid-1950's were interesting. Mortality ascribed to CHD was very low, although the Dutch were pictured as growing fat on a diet high in saturated fats; after all, the Netherlands has long been a major producer of butter fat, and the national breakfast is supposed to include cheese, eggs, and sausage as well as lots of butter.[40]

There are wide regional variations in diet and disease distribution in France with eight different dietary regions including the Mediterranean region of south-east France.[41]

According to a paper in the *Dialogues of Medicine*,[42] the French paradox is indeed a myth.

• • • • •

Teicholz states, "As it turns out, Dr Keys visited Crete during an unrepresentative period of extreme hardship after World War II." In addition to the preliminary survey in 1957, there were three rounds of surveys in Crete in 1960, 1965 and 1970 that were many years after the end of World War II. Keys did not work isolation. He worked with teams that included native speaking researchers. Keys was not in Crete for the first round of surveys in 1960 and was present only as an observer in 1970.

According to Teicholz:

> I found one of the most stunning and troubling errors. In that country, Keys had sampled the diets on Crete and Corfu more than once, in different seasons, in order to capture variations in the food eaten. Yet in an astonishing oversight, one of the three surveys on Crete fell during the forty-eight-day fasting period of Lent.

Teicholz claims she has uncovered a "stunning and troubling error". It was the local collaborators, Christ Aravanis and Andy Dontas and their colleagues, who carried out the surveys in Greece—not Ancel Keys, as stated by Teicholz. The Greek researchers were well aware of dietary regimes of the Greek Orthodox Church.

> The seasonal comparisons in Crete and Corfu were of interest because the survey in Crete in February and part of the survey in Corfu in March-April were in the 40-day fasting period of Lent of the Greek Orthodox Church, but strict adherence did not seem to be common in the populations of the present study.

Performing the dietary surveys during Lent was not a mistake or astonishing oversight. Teicholz states that the survey in question was during the 48-day fasting period of Lent —Lent is a 40-day period. Another point to consider is that the Orthodox Church specifies dietary restrictions for 180-200 days each year—not only for the 40-day period of Lent so the period of fasting during Lent is not as significant as suggested.

More than 95% of the eligible population participated in the survey. Keys and Henry Blackburn stated a number of times that they were studying the health of populations and that within those populations there could be a large variation with individuals.

• • • • •

David Kritchevsky (1920–2006) was a leading researcher relating to diet, nutrition and health. Teicholz states that Kritchevsky told her that "we were jumped on" when he suggested loosening the restrictions on dietary fat. Kritchevsky, however, did not deny the importance of raised blood cholesterol relating to both heart disease and cancer.

Kritchevsky did extensive work that showed animal protein raised cholesterol and caused more heart disease than a diet containing plant protein. He discovered that "in general, protein of animal origin is more cholesterolemic and atherogenic than plant protein."[43] He showed that a diet with a higher ratio of two amino acids (lysine to arginine ratio) raised cholesterol and produced more lesions. Lysine is more prevalent in animal protein.

He was involved in research that showed probucol and lovastatin (cholesterol-lowering drugs) were effective against atherogenesis.[44]

In 1954, he was the first to recognize that diets rich in saturated fatty acids were more atherogenic for rabbits than those with unsaturated fatty acids. Prior to this researchers were concentrating on total fat in the diet.

Kritchevsky co-authored a book *Cholesterol* (1958) and *Sitosterol* (1981) with OJ Pollak. Sitosterol is a cholesterol-like substance found in plants.

He partnered with Denis Burkitt in establishing the importance of dietary fiber in the diet and its relationship to colon cancer and other health issues that "challenged the dogma that fiber was inert, indigestible material."[45]

Kritchevsky's work does not support the hypothesis that cholesterol, saturated fats and animal proteins are irrelevant to heart disease.

• • • • •

Teicholz states that both the Inuit and Maasai are examples of healthy populations that thrive on a high-fat diet.

The foundations of the Inuit diet were fish (flesh and intestines), caribou meat, blubber, liver (seal and caribou), frozen deer droppings, and lichen obtained from caribou stomach. Meat was cached that was later retrieved, in varying stages of decay. Although men did eat raw meat during a hunt, Inuits did rely on a cooked, evening meal.[46] Carbohydrates are available in meat and liver in the form of glycogen.

Frozen mummies from the time before Western contact showed that Inuits suffered from osteoporosis, parasites including toxoplasma (caused by a parasitic protozoa) and trichinosis (caused by the larvae of roundworms), atherosclerosis, spina bifida, cribra orbitalia (spongy and porous bones in the skull), and iron deficiency.[47] [48] Spina bifida is associated with a lack of folic acid, which is found in cereals, grains, beans, and green leaves. Parasitic infections lower blood cholesterol. Inuit also suffer from a high rate of cerebral hemorrhage (a type of stroke) caused by a high level of oils obtained from fish that decreases the blood platelet clotting ability.[49]

Severe anthracosis has been found in female mummies. Anthracosis is caused by the accumulation of soot in due to prolonged exposure to smoky, seal-oil lamps.[50]

Similarly, Teicholz cites the Maasai as a healthy population that had a high meat diet. She quotes the work of George Mann, a doctor and medical researcher from Harvard and Vanderbilt Universities. Mann was a vocal critic of the diet-heart relationship. He believed that fit and active people are spared the complication of atherosclerosis.

According to Teicholz, Mann found that "he could identify almost no heart disease at all" in the Maasai.[51] Mann's paper, *Atherosclerosis in the Masai*, stated, "Measurements of the aorta showed extensive atherosclerosis with lipid infiltration and fibrous changes but very few complicated lesions. The coronary arteries showed intimal thickening by atherosclerosis which equaled that of old U.S. men."[52]

Maasai also have a very low energy intake in the foods, are active and suffer from parasitic infections—all which contribute to low serum cholesterol and lower the risk of heart disease.

• • • • •

Teicholz states that Henry Blackburn describes Keys as being "direct to the point of bluntness, critical to the point of skewering, and possessing a very quick, bright intelligence." The actual quote from Blackburn is "Ancel Keys has a quick and brilliant mind, a prodigious energy, and great perseverance. He can also be frank to the point of bluntness, and critical to the point of sharpness."[53]

Blackburn's words of "can be" has been transformed into "as being". Henry Blackburn and many other collaborators worked with Keys for decades. They held reunions. Margaret Keys was an essential collaborator in their work. Demonizing Keys is another strategy employed to discount his work.

• • • • •

Teicholz describes cholesterol as being "yellow"—it is white.

She also states, "The oils from linseed and rapeseed, in a genetically modified form, are blended to make "canola" oil. The "can" in canola is named for its origin, in Canada." It did originate in Canada in the 1970s. This is before the time of genetically modified foods or organisms. It was "developed by researchers from Agriculture and Agri-Food Canada and the University of Manitoba in the 1970s, using traditional plant breeding techniques."[54] It was bred from rapeseed, which is a *Brassica*, the genus which includes cabbages, kale, broccoli, and Brussel sprouts—linseed is not involved.

• • • • •

From the introduction of *The Big Fat Surprise*, Teicholz asserts:

> Unaware of the flimsy scientific scaffolding upon which their dietary guidelines rest, Americans

have dutifully attempted to follow them. Since the 1970s, we have successfully increased our fruits and vegetables by 17 percent, our grains by 29 percent, and reduced the amount of fat we eat from 43 percent to 33 percent of calories or less.

The claim from low-carb advocates that we have followed the low-fat guidelines for decades is ill-informed. A population consuming an average of 33% of calories of fat is not a low fat diet—10% of the population is consuming a diet with 40% fat or greater. Whilst the percentage of energy obtain from fat has decreased, the total amount of fat has increased as people are consuming more.

Whilst total vegetable consumption has increased 26%, this figure includes *potatoes for freezing* (that is, potato chips for frying) which increased 60% during the period. Fried potato chips does not really count as a vegetable.

From the conclusion of *The Big Fat Surprise*, Teicholz proclaims:

> The advice that comes out of this book is that a higher-fat diet is almost assuredly healthier in every way than one low in fat and high in carbohydrates. [...]

> Moreover, we now know that there are many good reasons to eat animal foods like red meat, cheese, eggs, and whole milk: they are particularly dense in nutrients— far more so than fruits and vegetables. [...]

And after all, red meat, cheese, and cream are delicious! Not to mention eggs fried in butter, cream sauces, and the drippings from a pan of roasted meats.

Teicholz is a passionate advocate of Dr Robert Atkins and his low-carbohydrate diet.

3

Common Myths

The U.S. has been consuming a low-fat diet for decades

The U.S. Department of Agriculture (USDA) issued the first dietary guidelines[55] in 1980, following the release of the second edition of the *McGovern Report*[56] in December, 1977. Included in the seven guidelines was the advice to "avoid too much fat, saturated fat, and cholesterol."

An argument that is made by many low-carbohydrate articles, books, and websites is that, despite following the expert medical advice to reduce fats for decades, we are fatter than ever. Many of popular articles claim that there is a conspiracy to hide the truth concerning fat and cholesterol.

However, USDA's Economic Research Service data suggests:

> [The] average daily calorie intake increased by 24.5 percent, or about 530 calories, between 1970 and 2000. Of that 24.5-percent increase, grains (mainly refined grain products) contributed 9.5 percentage points; added fats and oils, 9.0

percentage points; added sugars, 4.7 percentage points; fruits and vegetables together, 1.5 percentage points; meats and nuts together, 1 percentage point; and dairy products and eggs together, -1.5 percentage point.[57]

Since the low point of 1957–1958, total food consumption to the year 2000 has increased 24.5% from 2170 calories to 2700 calories.

The plate-size and serving-size has increased over the past several decades. As a result, the total calories consumed also rose significantly by 24%.[58]

The same publication shows the increase in different food groups since the 1950s. Note that the table below shows the weight of the food items. Fats and oils are more energy-dense than carbohydrates and proteins. They contain more than twice the energy found in the same weight of carbohydrates and proteins. Whilst the percentage of calories derived from fat has reduced from approximately 40% of total calories to 33%, the total amount of calories and total amount of fats has actually increased.

Item	1950–1959	1970–1979	2000	% change 1950s–2000
Total Meats	138.2	177.2	195.2	41
Poultry	20.5	35.2	66.5	224
Fish	10.9	12.5	15.2	39
All dairy	703	548	593	-16
Cheese	7.7	14.4	29.8	287
Milk	36.4	29.8	24.3	-33
Added Fats and Oils	44.6	53.4	74.5	67
Total Calorific Sweeteners (sugars)	109.6	123.7	152.4	39

U.S. per Capita Annual Average (lbs)

The amount of total meats, poultry, fish, added fats and oils, and calorific sweeteners (sugars) have increased since the 1950s, which is decades prior to the first dietary guidelines being published. After a decrease in dairy and cheese consumption from 1950s to 1970s, these items have since increased. Egg consumption is also rising after reaching a low in the 1990s.

Whilst the consumption of grain products have increased, the increase is a result of consuming highly-processed refined flours. As a result, "consumers eat too much refined grain, too little whole grain."

Heart disease is caused by sugar consumption

The proponents of the low-carbohydrate diet contend that the real cause of heart disease is sugar. Frequently, all carbohydrates are made the villain—not just sugar.

John Yudkin was a passionate advocate of the theory that has been taken up by a number of recent commentators. Yudkin noticed that sugar consumption increased more than any other food component of the last century and was closely correlated with the increase in cardiovascular disease.

Yudkin published the book *Pure, White and Deadly: the problem with sugar*[59] in 1972. This book did not contain any references. His popular books and campaigning through the media weakened the medical positions on heart disease. Mortality from heart disease started reducing in 1966 in U.S., Finland, and Australia. It was another 10 years before this happened in the United Kingdom because of Yudkin's influence.[60]

Geoffrey Rose believed that there would have been 25,000 fewer deaths in England and Wales if the gains made in Australia and America were duplicated in the United Kingdom.[61]

Some reasons for dismissing the association of sugar consumption with heart disease include:

- Sucrose does not ordinarily raise plasma cholesterol.
- If starch is replaced in the diet with sucrose then plasma triglycerides are not increased.
- There is no mechanism where sucrose could lead to heart disease.
- Countries such as Costa Rica, Cuba, and Venezuela have high sugar consumption but low rates of heart disease.

- Keys's *Seven Countries Study* did show a strong correlation with the percentage of dietary calories supplied by sucrose and heart disease, with the correlation of 0.78. The correlation of percentage of calories supplied by saturated fatty acids and heart disease is even greater at 0.86. Since there was a strong correlation (0.84) between sucrose and saturated fatty acids in the countries studied, this explains the high correlation with sucrose consumption and heart disease.[62]
- The consumption of sugar was much greater in Sweden than in neighboring Finland, but the age-specific cardiovascular death rate in Sweden is not much more than half that in Finland.[63]

Heart disease is caused by wheat consumption

According to some low-carbohydrate diet advocates, wheat consumption is another possibility for the cause of heart disease.

The *China-Cornell-Oxford Project* did correlate wheat-flour consumption with an increase rate of cardiovascular diseases. However, an increase in wheat-flour consumption was also correlated to lower green-vegetable consumption, a higher consumption of meat-based diets, lower serum levels of monounsaturated fats (such as olive oil), and a higher body weight. All these factors are associated with a higher risk of heart disease.

A review, published in *The Journal of Nutrition*[64], of 45 prospective cohort studies and 21 randomized-controlled trials between 1966 and February 2012 found that an increase in the intake of whole grain foods is associated with *lower* risk of type 2 diabetes, cardiovascular disease, and weight gain.

The conclusion of the paper is that "this meta-analysis provide evidence to support beneficial effects of whole-grain intake on vascular disease prevention."

Heart disease is caused by pumping of blood

Dr Ernest Curtis proposes that heart disease is caused by hydraulic stress of the blood pumping through arteries. Curtis states that since cholesterol is found throughout the circulatory system then lesions should be found in both arteries and veins—not just in the branch points in the arteries.

In the second decade of the twentieth century, Nikolaj Anitschkow had determined "that the earliest lesions, caused by a high cholesterol diet, occurred at the root of the aorta and in the aortic arch. The location of these lesion was most likely determined by hemodynamic factors".[65]

We are looking at two independent observations—the observation that cholesterol is involved in the formation of lesions and the lesions are located in places that are determined by fluid dynamics. Both observations can be true.

Coconut oil is a health food

Coconut oil is passionately advocated as a wonderful product that has a multitude of health benefits.

> The health benefits of coconut oil include hair care, skin care, stress relief, cholesterol level maintenance, weight loss, boosted immune system, proper digestion, and regulated metabolism. It also provides relief from kidney problems, heart diseases, high blood pressure, diabetes, HIV, and cancer, while helping to improve dental quality and bone strength.[66]

Fats contain 2¼ times more calories than the same weight of carbohydrates. They are not as filling so you can eat more.

All fats damage the endothelial lining of the arteries—cells cannot produce nitric oxide.

Coconut oil contains over 85% of saturated fat. It is higher in saturated fats than lard or butter. Saturated fats increases the viscosity of blood, increases risk of thrombosis, increases the stickiness (adhesiveness) of blood cells, and damages the endothelial lining of the arteries.

Not all saturated fats raise cholesterol levels. Only lauric acid, myristic acid, and palmitic acid causes an increase in cholesterol. Of all the oils, coconut oil contains the most (over 66%) of the above fatty acids. Coconut oil does raise cholesterol.[67] [68] [69]

Cholesterol helps fight infections and inflammation

Headlines occasionally appear on the internet and popular magazines that argue high cholesterol helps fight infections. Some examples are:

- It's well known that cholesterol helps fight infections.
- High cholesterol may be helping you fight off disease and inflammation.
- Does high cholesterol help us fight our infections?
- Cholesterol may help fight infections.

The mechanism for achieving this is not usually stated although articles suggest that the anti-oxidant properties of cholesterol may be responsible.

A paper published in 2012 details the mechanism how *lowered* cholesterol protects against viral infection.[70]

Lowering cholesterol causes cancer and depression

The claim that lowering cholesterol increases the risk of depression, suicide, and cancer appears to have originated from the *Multiple Risk Factor Intervention Trial* (MRFIT).

The study followed 361,662 U.S. men. After 6 years, the study showed that the total mortality reached a low point with serum cholesterol at approximately 180 mg/dL (4.7 mmol/L).[71] Mortality increased as cholesterol levels fell below 4.7 mmol/L.

A number of factors influence serum cholesterol—not only diet. Parasitic infections, liver disease, a number of cancers, and infectious disease cause weight loss and a decrease in serum cholesterol. It is illness that has an impact on emotional well-being.

The fact that mortality and cholesterol levels lower than 4.7 mmol/dL are negatively correlated does not mean that low cholesterol causes a higher mortality. A person may lose weight and cholesterol levels fall because of sickness.

The *China-Cornell-Oxford Project* showed a decrease in serum cholesterol correlated with a decrease in the mortality rate. The lowest average cholesterol levels were 80 mg/dL (2.1 mmol/L) for females and 95 mg/dL (2.5 mmol/L) for males in a xiang (village) in the Sichuan province located in central China. This was not associated with an increase in mortality.

Low cholesterol leads to low vitamin D and sex hormones

One argument is that if our cholesterol is too low then we are unable to manufacture sufficient vitamin D and sex hormones.

Lack of vitamin D is associated with colon, breast, and prostate cancer, osteoporosis, multiple sclerosis, type I diabetes, heart disease, mental illness, muscle weakness and coordination, obesity, and osteoarthritis so it is essential that we do not jeopardize our ability to produce it.

Also, we would not be wanting to do anything that inhibits the production of the sex hormones. Since cholesterol is a precursor of testosterone, estrogen, progesterone, cortisol, and vitamin D, as well as bile acids, then the argument is presented that too little cholesterol will result in insufficient quantities of the resulting products.

Firstly, this is presented as a fact, without any evidence to back it up.

Secondly, vitamin D and hormones are required in the smallest quantities—much, much smaller than the quantity of cholesterol that our bodies produce. Each liter of blood contains approximately 1.5 to 2.5 grams of cholesterol. (Three garden peas weigh about a gram.) There is over 100 grams of cholesterol in adults.

Hormones are required in smallest of quantities. Below is a guide to the units used to measure the concentrations of steroids in the blood.

Steroid	Examples	Notes
25-hydoxycholecalciferol (vitamin D3)	40 mg/L	milli – thousands
Cortisol	120 µg/L	micro – millionths
Progesterone	10 µg/L	
Testosterone (male)	5.2 µg/L	
Aldosterone	122 ng/L	nano - billionths
Estradiol	250 ng/L	

There does not appear to be any evidence that low cholesterol reduces the ability of the body to produce the sterol hormones.

Sugar (or Carbohydrate) causes cancer

A view that is prevalent in the popular press is that sugar causes cancer and should be avoided. A number of doctors, dietitians, and naturopaths hold this view. Since starches are digested as simple sugars then it is recommended that starches should also be avoided.

As a result, a low-carbohydrate diet is endorsed. Some practitioners recommend high levels of vegetables that are high in nutrients but low in the amount of energy that is provided. The absence of starch from these diets results in a calorie-restricted diet that is possibly ketogenic. If a diet is restricted in carbohydrates, it will be high in fat and protein. Ketogenic diets are difficult to maintain.

Ketosis occurs when fat in the body is utilized to obtain energy in the absence of glucose. Glucose is normally obtained from the digestion of carbohydrates. Ketosis results in the production of ketones—acetone being one of the three types of ketones produced during ketosis. Blood acidity rises with an increase in ketones.

Serious complications with a ketogenic diet have been reported, even when performed under medical supervision. These issues relate to the high levels of protein and include a lack of appetite, headaches, nausea, acidosis, and hypoproteinemia.[72]

• • • • •

Epidemiological studies comparing diet and rates of cancers have failed to show a link between carbohydrate intake and the rate of common cancers such as breast, prostate, colon, and rectal cancers.

Ken Carroll of University of Western Ontario (Canada) studied that components of the diet and the incidence of cancers in more than 30 countries.[73][74] These studies showed a strong correlation with the prevalence of a number of cancers (breast, prostate, intestinal, leukemia, rectal and pancreatic cancers), and the amount of fat in the diet.

Similarly, the *China-Cornell-Oxford Project* studied 65 counties in China. This showed a positive correlation between the amount of animal source foods and the levels of breast, prostate, colon, and rectal cancers. The consumption of animal source foods and the prevalence of these cancers is much less than in the U.S.

• • • • •

A distinction must be made between added sugars consumed in isolation and carbohydrates that are consumed as part of a whole-food diet. Adding table sugar (sucrose) that is obtained from sugar cane and sugar beets to our diets is not beneficial to our health. High-fructose corn syrup is another added sugar commonly found in processed food that has detrimental health benefits.

Cancer cells consume more glucose than normal cells but this does not imply that removing all sugars and carbohydrates from your diet will benefit cancer outcomes.

A study[75] published in 2012 investigated the effects of different types of sugars in the diet and their effect on cancer. This study investigated the association of total sugars, sucrose, fructose, added sugars, added sucrose, and added fructose in the diet with the risk of 24 malignancies.

435,674 participants aged 50–71 years were followed for seven years. These sugars were not associated with an increased risk of colorectal, breast, prostate, pancreatic, endometrial cancers, or with other IGF-1 related cancers. Insulin-like growth factor-1 (IGF-1) is a hormone that promotes the growth of tissues, including cancer cells.

All sugars studied were inversely associated with risk of ovarian cancer—the more sugar consumed then the risk of ovarian cancer was reduced.

There was an increased risk with some relatively rare cancers such as esophageal adenocarcinoma, pleural cancer, and small intestinal cancers. The researchers suggested the "possibility of chance results" for this finding because of the low incidence of these cancers.

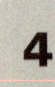

4

The Basics

What are Fats?

Fats and oils are a chemical combination of three fatty acids joined by glycerol—hence the term *triglycerides*.

Chemical compounds are represented by a diagram of its chemical structure. Hydrogen, oxygen, nitrogen, and carbon usually have 1, 2, 3, and 4 bonds respectively connecting them to other elements. One exception to this is when carbon forms rings as in benzene. A benzene consists molecule consists of 6 carbon and 6 hydrogen. Below is a diagram showing the structure of ethane and ethylene (ethene).

Chemical structure of ethane and ethylene

A double bond between two carbon atoms is indicated by a double line.

Fatty acids consist of a chain of carbon and hydrogen atoms with a carboxyl group at one end. The carboxyl group is frequently represented as -COOH. The carboxyl group consists of two chemical groups: the carbonyl group (-C=O); and the hydroxyl group (-O-H).

Most fatty acids have 4 to 28 carbon atoms with an even number of carbon atoms. The number of carbon atoms and the number and position of the double bonds define the type of fatty acid.

The letters C and H representing carbon and hydrogen atoms are often omitted from the diagrams. Since carbon have four bonds and hydrogen has one bond, the presence of these atoms can be deduced.

Fatty acid chains are characterized by length.

- Short-chain fatty acids are fatty acids with 6 or less carbon atoms.
- Medium-chain fatty acids are fatty acids with 7 to 12 carbons atoms.
- Long-chain fatty acids are fatty acids with tails 13 to 22 carbons.
- Very long chain fatty acids are fatty acids with tails longer than 22 carbons.

Saturated Fatty Acids

Saturated fatty acids do not have any double bonds between the carbon atoms. Saturated fats have a higher melting point and are more likely to be solid. Animal fats usually have a greater saturated fat content. They are more chemically stable and are less likely to go rancid.

For example, lauric acid.

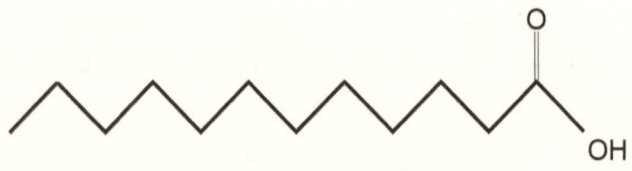

Lauric acid

Unsaturated Fatty Acids

Unsaturated fatty acids have at least one double bound. Unsaturated fats have a lower melting point and are more likely to be liquid. Vegetable fats usually are higher in unsaturated fats and are more likely to go rancid.

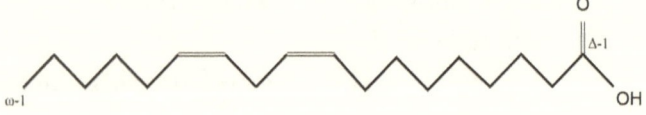

Linoleic acid

Cis-Fatty Acids and Trans-Fatty Acids

Oleic and elaidic fatty acids have the same number of atoms—both have one double bond in the same position. The carbon atoms that have the double bond have only one hydrogen atom attached. Oleic acid has the hydrogen atoms on the same side of the molecule making it a *cis*-fatty acid (pronounced as *sis*, meaning *on the same side*). Elaidic acid has the hydrogen atoms on the opposite side making it a *trans*-fatty acid (meaning *on the opposite side* or *across*).

Oleic acid - a cis-fatty acid

Elaidic acid - a trans-fatty acid

A cis-fatty acid is bent at the double bond, whereas the trans-fatty acid is straight.

If a fatty acid has more than one double bond, then each double bond is either *trans* or *cis*.

Trans-fats are primarily produced by frying or by hydrogenation. By adding hydrogen atoms to unsaturated fats to eliminate the double bonds may cause the formation of trans-fats. If all the double bonds are eliminated then a saturated fatty acid is produced. Otherwise, a trans-fatty acid may be formed.

There are three main reasons why trans-fatty acids are detrimental to our health.

- Compared with unsaturated fatty acids, trans-fatty acids increase total cholesterol, LDL cholesterol and triglycerides. Trans-fatty acids also decrease HDL cholesterol, which is considered to be a disadvantage. Saturated fatty acids raise total cholesterol and LDL cholesterol more than trans-fatty acids. Saturated fatty-acids also raise HDL cholesterol.[76] The risk of cardiovascular disease with trans-fats is greater than expected based on only changes to the lipid profile.[77]
- Trans-fatty acid intake is associated with an increased level of biomarkers of inflammation and endothelial dysfunction. Endothelial cells line the surface of blood and lymphatic vessels.
- Fatty acids are components of cell membranes. Trans-fatty acids are straight molecules and cis-fatty acids are bent at the double bond. As a result, the fluidity of the cell membranes is decreased and the permeability is increased with an increase of trans-fatty acids.[78]

Conjugated linoleic acids (CLAs) are found in dairy products. The unsaturated carbon atoms of CLAs are separated by one carbon atom instead of the normal two carbon atoms.

Vaccenic and rumenic acids are the main trans-fatty acids found in dairy. They are both sold as health products.

According to the National Academies of Sciences:

> Trans fatty acids are not essential and provide no known benefit to human health. [...] A UL [Upper Limit] is not set for trans fatty acids because any incremental increase in trans fatty acid intake increases CHD risk. Because trans fatty acids are unavoidable in ordinary, non-vegan diets, consuming 0 percent of energy would require significant changes in patterns of dietary intake. [...] Nevertheless, it is recommended that trans fatty acid consumption be as low as possible while consuming a nutritionally adequate diet.[79]

Whilst suggesting that we consume no trans-fatty acids, the report deems that it is not practical.

Naming of Fatty Acids

There are a number of different naming conventions for fatty acids.

With the omega-numbering system, the numbering of the carbon atoms commences at the opposite end to where the carboxyl group is located—omega being the last letter of the Greek alphabet. Therefore, an omega-3 fatty acid has its first double bond at the third-last carbon atom. This is denoted by n-3 or ω-3.

Other symbols used to describe fatty acids are the C:D numbers that denote the number of carbon atoms and the number of double bonds.

The delta (Δ) naming system describes each double bond. Each double bond is described as *cis* or *trans* followed by Δ with the position of the saturated carbon atom. The counting of the carbon atoms commences from the carboxyl group end, which differs from the omega-numbering system. For example, rumenic acid is described as 18:2 *cis, trans*-Δ^9, Δ^{11}. Alternatively, it may be denoted by 18:2 *cis-9, trans-11*.

Below are some examples of fatty acids.

Butyric acid	4:0	Butyric acid is found in milk, butter and cheese.
Caproic acid	6:0	Caproic acid is found in small amounts in the milk of mammals, particularly cows, goats and sheep.
Caprylic acid	8:0	Caprylic acid is found in the milk of mammals, particularly goats and sheep. It also occurs in coconut oil.
Capric acid	10:0	Capric acid occurs in coconut oil and palm kernel oil. It also occurs in milk of mammals, particularly goats and sheep.

Lauric acid	12:0	Lauric acid is a major component of coconut oil, laurel oil (from the Mediterranean Bay Tree) and palm kernel oil. It is also found in human breast milk (6% of total fat), cow's milk (3%) and goat's milk (3%).
Myristic acid	14:0	Myristic acid is found in nutmeg, palm kernel oil, coconut oil, butter fat and is a minor component of many animal fats.
Palmitic acid	16:0	Palmitic acid is the most common fatty acid found in both plants and animals. It is a major component of the oil from palm trees (palm oil, palm kernel oil and coconut oil), meats, cheeses, butter, and dairy products.
Stearic acid	18:0	Second most common fatty acid. Occurs in animal fats up to 30% and vegetable fats is usually less than 5%. It is, however, a large component of cocoa butter and shea butter.
Palmitoleic acid	16:1 n-7 cis-9	Palmitoleic acid is found in animal tissues as well as palm oil, coconut oil, and macadamia oil.
Oleic acid	18:1 n-9 cis-9	Occurs in both animal and vegetable fats. It is a large component of olive oil.
Linoleic acid LA	18:2 n-6 cis-9, cis-12	Linoleic acid is found in many seed oils such as poppy seed, safflower, sunflower, vegetable oils, nuts, and corn. With a normal diet, more than adequate amount of linoleic acid is available. It is an omega-6 fatty acid. This is one of the two essential fatty acids for humans.

α–linolenic acid ALA	18:3 n-3 cis-9, cis-12, cis-15	α–linolenic is found in many leafy green vegetables such as brassicas, spinach, and lettuce. It is also found in walnuts and fish oils. It is an omega-3 fatty acid. This is one of the two essential fatty acids for humans.
γ–linolenic acid GLA	18:3 n-6 cis-6, cis-9, cis-12	γ–linolenic found in canola, soybeans, walnuts, chia, evening primrose, and flaxseed. It is an omega-6 fatty acid.
Arachidonic acid AA	20:4 n-6 cis-5, cis-8, cis-11, cis-14	Arachidonic acid is a polyunsaturated fatty acid present in the phospholipids of membranes of the body's cells and is abundant in the brain, muscles, and liver. Humans can synthesis AA from linoleic acid (LA). It is an omega-6 fatty acid.
Eicosapentaenoic acid EPA	20:5 n-3 cis-5, cis-8, cis-11, cis-14, cis-17	This appears to be essential for brain development in the young of mammals. It is found in fish oil and in the milk of mammals. After weaning, it is synthesized by mammals from α-linolenic acid (ALA). It is an omega-3 fatty acid.
Docosahexaenoic acid DHA	22:6 n-3 cis-4, cis-7, cis-10, cis-13, cis-16, cis-19	It is a major component of the human brain. Cold-water fish are rich in DHA, which is obtained from algae. It is found in the milk of mammals. After weaning, it is synthesized by mammals from α-linolenic acid (ALA). It is an omega-3 fatty acid.

Elaidic acid	18:1 n-9 trans-9	Elaidic acid is the major trans-fatty acid found in margarines, which are hydrogenated vegetables oils. It is the trans-fatty acid variant (isomer) of oleic acid.
Vaccenic acid	18:1 n-7 trans-11	Vaccenic acid is the main trans-fatty acid found in dairy products and the fats of ruminants. The cis-version of vaccenic acid is relatively rare and found in sea-buckthorn—a genus containing seven species of deciduous shrubs found in Europe and Asia.
Rumenic acid	18:2 n-7 cis-9, trans-11	Rumenic acid is the main conjugated linoleic acid (CLA), which is found in dairy and in the fat of cows and other ruminants. It is a trans-fatty acid.

Triglycerides and Phospholipids

Triglycerides are the main components of vegetable oils and animal fats. It is formed by combining three fatty acids molecules with a glycerol molecule.

Phospholipids are a major component of all cell membranes. They usually contain two fatty acids and a phosphate group. Other chemical groups, such as choline or inositol, can be attached to the phosphate group. Lecithin is a phospholipid that is found in egg yolk. Lecithin contains choline.

A normal cell membrane is made up of two layers of phospholipid molecules that normally comprises of cis-fatty acids. As we have seen, these fatty acid molecules are bent at the double bonds—the more double bonds, the more bends. Introduce trans-fats and unsaturated fats, which are straight molecules, then cell membrane permeability and fluidity are affected.

Omega-6 to Omega-3 Ratio

During most of human evolution, the ratio of omega-6 to omega-3 fatty acid was about 1:1. With increase production of grains, which have a higher omega-6 fatty acid content, the ratio has increased—the ratio is now 10:1 to 25:1.

The usual solution is to increase the intake of omega-3 by eating flaxseed oil or fish oil. A healthier alternative is to decrease the amount of fat and omega-6 intake.

Healthy Oils

There are many studies that suggest that "healthy oils" do not have any health benefits and actually increase health risks.

A review of 48 random clinical trials and 41 cohort studies was published in 2006. It showed, "Long chain and shorter chain omega-3 fats do not have a clear effect on total mortality, combined cardiovascular events or cancer."[80]

An article published in 2007 concluded, "These findings provide evidence that associations observed in studies suggesting a benefit of fish or long-chain ω-3 FAs [fatty acids] may be due to a convergence of greater fish intakes with an overall healthier dietary pattern rather than with a specific effect of long-chain ω-3 FAs."[81]

Blood thinning properties of omega-3 fats that prevent the formation of clots also increases the chance of bleeding complications such as cerebral hemorrhage.[82]

What are Proteins?

Proteins are chains made of amino acids linked together. Our bodies cannot use proteins directly. The proteins are broken down into their amino acid constituents in the stomach by enzymes. There are 21 amino acids that are the building blocks of proteins. 9 of these must be provided in the food we eat. The others can be synthesized by our bodies.[83]

Some of the functions of proteins are listed below:

- Most enzymes are proteins. They are involved in chemical reactions that take place in cells. For example, enzymes such as amylases and proteases break down starch and proteins into their constituent components so the intestines can absorb them.
- Some hormones are proteins that transmit signals to coordinate biological processes between different cells and organs. For example, growth hormones and insulin.
- Antibodies bind to specific foreign particles, such as viruses and bacteria, to help protect the body.

- Structural proteins include keratins (skin, fur, hair, wool, claws, nails, hooves, horns, scales, beaks, and feathers), actin and myosin proteins found in muscle tissue, and collagens found in tendons.
- Proteins are used to bind and carry molecules within cells and throughout the body. For example, proteins are used to transport cholesterol in the blood.

Francois Magendie (1783–1855) was a professor of anatomy in Paris. He made a distinction between nitrogenous and non-nitrogenous components of foods. Protein is the only major component that contains nitrogen.

Gerritt Mulder was born in the Netherlands and earned a medical degree from Utrecht University. He described the chemical composition of protein and was the first to use the name, protein, in a publication, in 1838 paper *'On the composition of some animal substances'*. In the same publication he also proposed that animals draw most of their protein from plants. The word protein is from the Greek word: proteios, "the first quality" or "of prime importance."[84]

Carl von Voit was a professor in Germany. He has been referred to as the Father of Nutrition. He was a mentor of many prominent nutrition researchers. After studying laborers, who consumed approximately 3,100 Calories daily, Voit concluded that protein intake for people should be 118 grams per day. He believed that people with sufficient income to afford almost any choice of foods—from meat to vegetables—would instinctively select an optimum diet.

One of his students was Wilbur Atwater (1844–1907). He was a prominent and influential American nutritionist at the end of the 1800s. He originated the systematic chemical analysis of foods in the United States. He and his co-workers established the caloric values of protein, fat, and carbohydrate, taking into account digestibility and compiled nutrient tables of thousands of items of food. He helped start and manage the system of federally-funded agricultural experimental stations.[85]

Since protein is the only major food group that contains nitrogen, it is possible to determine the protein requirements by examining the nitrogen balance in the body. You cannot store protein so any excess protein is broken down into ammonia, which is converted to urea and eliminated from the body. You do not build muscles by eating additional protein.

Atwater showed that the maintenance of nitrogen equilibrium was possible at levels little above one-third of the Voit Standard. Atwater reported, "Men with more or less activity have maintained nitrogen equilibrium on 7 g of nitrogen or 44 g protein per day."[86] He did not feel that these observations justified lowering the standard protein intake requirements.

After completing one study in the early 1900s, Atwater concluded, "Americans consumed too much fat and sweets and did not exercise enough."

Russell Henry Chittenden was professor of physiological chemistry at Yale from 1882 to 1922. He was not convinced that the Voit Standard protein requirement was correct. As Chittenden explained:

> Fats and carbohydrates when oxidized in the body are ultimately burned to simple gaseous products.
>
> [Proteid foods] when oxidized, yield a row of crystalline nitrogenous products which ultimately pass out of the body through the kidneys—frequently spoken of as toxins—float about through the body and may exercise more or less of a deleterious influence upon the system, or, being temporarily deposited, may exert some specific or local influence that calls for their speedy removal.[87]

He reduced his own protein intake from 150 grams a day to around 40 grams a day. He lost weight and become healthier.

He repeated the experiment on five sedentary Yale staff (62 g protein per day), then thirteen members of the Army Corps of Engineers (61 g protein per day) who were physically fit and active. Finally, eight Yale Olympic-class athletes repeated the experiment consuming an average of 64 g protein per day. They improved their performance by 30-35% and maintained a positive protein balance—that is, they consumed more protein than they lost.

The nutrient reference values of protein for Australia and New Zealand[88] are shown below.

g/(kg · day)	Age
1.43	infants: 0–6 months
1.60	infants: 7–12 months
1.08	1–3 years
0.91	4–8 years
0.94 0.99	9–13 years (male) 9–13 years (female)
0.87 0.77	14–18 years (male) 14–18 years (female)
0.84 0.75	19–70 years (male) 19–70 years (female)
1.07 0.94	70+ years (male) 70+ years (female)
1.00	Secord and third trimester pregnancy, using pre-pregnancy weight
1.10	lactating women

The World Health Organization of the United Nations recommendations are slightly different.[89]

In human milk, approximately 5-7% of the calories are derived from protein. At the time when the need for protein is at its greatest, infants can thrive on a diet of only 7% or less of protein.

Many people, including dieticians and doctors, assume that the *Recommended Dietary Intake* (RDI) is the minimum amount of nutrient that we need.

The distribution of nutrient requirements for people often approximates a normal distribution. Most people have the average requirements with an equal number of people having a greater requirement and a smaller requirement.

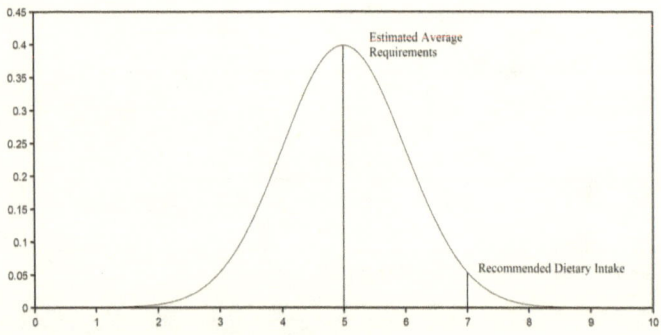

The deviation is the difference between the average measurement and an actual measurement. If the average is 5 and the value is 6 then the deviation is 1.

The standard deviation is a measure of how scattered the results are. A small standard deviation means that the results are clustered around the average. A large standard deviation means that the results of more widely scattered.

The standard deviation in the graph above is 1. The RDI is 2 standard deviations above the average requirement. The result is that the RDI meets or exceeds the requirements of at least 97.8% of the population.

The RDI for protein for a 76 kg male is 76 * 0.83 = 63 g protein.

Protein yields 4 kcalories / gram. Therefore, a diet of 2,900 kcalories with only 10% protein provides 2900 * 10% / 4 = 72 grams of protein which exceeds the RDI.[90]

Despite the RDI indicating that 98% of the population will meet or exceed their protein requirements at approximately 10% of the diet, the *Acceptable Macronutrient Distribution Range* (in Australia) for protein is set to 15-25% of calories consumption. Eating more protein than required is not beneficial—it is has a negative impact.

Plant-based foods contain relatively low amounts of the amino acids lysine, leucine, and methionine.

Note: A food calorie (Cal) is equal to 1000 scientific calories. The USDA Nutrition Database lists the energy value of foods in units of 1000 scientific calories (kcal). A scientific calorie is the energy required to raise the temperature of 1 gram of water by 1ºC at standard atmospheric pressure.

Therefore, when dealing with nutrition, *calorie* and *kilocalorie* can refer to the same units.

What are Carbohydrates?

A carbohydrate is a compound that consists only of carbon, hydrogen, and oxygen. The ratio of hydrogen to oxygen atom is approximately 2:1—as in water.

Carbohydrates contain more than 90% of the dry matter of plants.

One way that carbohydrates can be grouped is into the following four categories:

- monosaccharides
- disaccharides
- oligosaccharides
- polysaccharides

Monosaccharides

Monosaccharides are carbohydrates that cannot be broken down to simpler carbohydrates. They are often referred to as simple sugars.

- Glucose occurs in its free form in plant tissues, fruits, honey and blood. In most natural foodstuffs glucose is present as a component of disaccharides and polysaccharides.
- Fructose is found in its free state in plant juices, fruit and honey. It is the sweetest sugar known in nature.
- Galactose does not occur in its free state in nature. It exists as a component of many polysaccharides.

Disaccharides

Disaccharides are composed of two simple sugars joined together.

- Maltose is composed of two molecules of glucose joined together. Maltose is found in sprouted wheat and barley. Maltose is the major sugar in beer.
- Sucrose is composed of one molecule of glucose and fructose joined together. Sucrose occurs widely in nature in most plants. Rich sources of sucrose include sugar cane (20% sucrose) and sugar beet (15–20%).
- Lactose is composed of one molecule of glucose and galactose joined together. Lactose, or milk sugar, is the principal sugar found in milk and is unique to mammals. It forms about 40% of the total milk solids. Lactose readily undergoes bacterial fermentation: for example, the souring of milk by *Streptococcus lactis* by the fermentation of lactose to lactic acid.

Oligosaccharides

Oligosaccharides comprise of two to ten monosaccharide or two to twenty monosaccharide units depending upon the author. This definition includes the disaccharides.

- Raffinose is a trisaccharide composed of galactose, fructose, and glucose. It can be found in beans, cabbage, Brussels sprouts, broccoli, asparagus, as well as other vegetables, and whole grains. Humans are lacking the enzyme to breakdown raffinose. Bacteria in the lower intestine ferment raffinose to carbon dioxide and methane leading to flatulence.
- Stachyose consists of four saccharides—two galactose and a glucose unit with a fructose unit. Stachyose is naturally found in numerous vegetables

(e.g. green beans, soybeans, and other beans) and plants. Stachyose is less sweet than sucrose and is used commercially as a sweetener. It is not completely digestible.

Polysaccharides

Polysaccharides are much larger than the oligosaccharides, containing hundreds or thousands of monosaccharide units. Some common food examples are listed below.

- Starch is composed of two structural components, amylose and amylopectin. The proportions vary depending upon the plant source varying from 20–30% for amylose and 70–80% for amylopectin. Both amylose and amylopectin consist of glucose. Starch occurs in stems, fruits, seeds, roots, and leaves. Starch is the predominant food reserve substance in plants and provides 70–80% of the calories consumed by humans world-wide.
- Glycogen is composed glucose units. Carbohydrates are stored within the animal body as glycogen. It is concentrated in the liver and muscles.
- Inulin is found in onion, garlic, asparagus, and bananas. The primary commercial source is chicory and Jerusalem artichoke tubers. Inulins are composed mainly of fructose units and usually have a terminal glucose. Inulin is not digested in the stomach or small intestine. It is a component of dietary fiber and has a beneficial effect by stimulating the growth of bacterial species already present in the colon. They do not raise

the glucose or the insulin levels in the blood. It is used as a filler in commercially produced products.

- Cellulose is composed of very long chains of glucose units. It is a very stable polysaccharide and is not digestible by humans.
- Gums are water-soluble polysaccharides that are constituents of plant wounds.
- Mucilages are present in seaweeds, some plants, and seeds. These are soluble in hot water and cool to a gel.
- Pectic substances are abundant in citrus fruit, sugar beet, apples, and some root vegetables such as turnips. They have gelling properties and are often used in the preparation of jams.

Dietary Fiber

Carbohydrates are the principal source of metabolic energy for humans and also the principal providers of the bulk and body of food products.

Cellulose, lignin, and pectin are components of dietary fiber. Other components of dietary fiber include non-digestible oligosaccharides such as raffinose and stachyose.

Only monosaccharides can be absorbed through the wall of the small intestine and only glucose is produced by digestion of polysaccharides in humans.

Dietary fiber is important in nutrition because it maintains the normal functioning of the gastrointestinal tract. Dietary fiber increases intestinal bulk, which accelerates intestinal transit time, and helps prevent constipation. Fiber decreases blood cholesterol levels and reduces the chances of colonic cancer.

Fiber and starches that have not been digested by the time they reach the large intestine are fermented by more than 400 species of bacteria. The result is short-chain fatty acids that provides some energy and is beneficial for colon health.

Type 2 Diabetes and Insulin Resistance

The result of Type 2 diabetes is that the body does not process sugar effectively, which results in high levels of glucose in the blood. High levels of glucose over an extended period of time places you at risk for many serious health problems.

The usual medical advice is to prescribe a diet with very little sugar and limit starch in the diet since glucose is formed as a result of starch being digested.

This does seem to be the logical solution to having too much glucose in the blood.

It has been known since at least 1927 that high fat diets increase insulin resistance.[91] [92] Healthy, young medical students were divided into four dietary groups:

- high-carbohydrate diet consisting of sugar, candy, syrup, baked potatoes, bananas, and oatmeal, rice, and white bread
- high-fat diet consisting of olive oil, butter, mayonnaise, egg-yolks, and cream

- high-protein diet consisting of lean meat, lean fish, and egg-whites
- the fourth group was placed on a fasting regime

The students were fed their diets for two days and a glucose tolerance test was performed on the morning of the third day.

The students who consumed the high-carbohydrate showed an increase in tolerance for dextrose; those on the high-protein diet showed a mild inability to remove sugar from the blood; those on the high-fat and starvation diets showed a significant decrease in their tolerance for sugar.

After only two days on their experimental diets, the only group showing a normal, healthy response to the glucose tolerance test was the high-carbohydrate group.

Normally, insulin attaches to protein receptors on the cell's surface and signals the cell membrane to allow glucose to enter. If there is an accumulation of fat in the cell, it interferes with insulin's signaling process and glucose cannot enter the cell. Fat can accumulate inside muscle cells even in slim people. The real cause of type 2 diabetes is not an excess of sugar or carbohydrates. It is an accumulation of fat inside the cells that interferes with the muscle cells' ability to respond to insulin. The muscle cells are unable to access glucose, which is required for energy production.

An intervention trial,[93] published in 2006, compared 99 individuals being treated for type 2 diabetes. 49 were placed on a low-fat vegan diet and 50 on a diet following the American Diabetes Association (ADA) diet. The results were compared after a 22 week period.

In every criteria measured, the participants in the low-fat vegan diet performed better than those following the ADA diet. The values shown are the average of the two groups.

Criteria	Vegan	ADA
% of participants that reduced diabetic medication	43%	23%
Reduction in HbA1C	0.96	0.56
Reduction in HbA1C (Excluding those who reduced medication)	1.23	0.38
Body weight decrease (kg)	6.5	3.1
LDL cholesterol decrease (%) (Excluding those who reduced medication)	21.2	10.7
Reduction in urinary albumin (mg/24 h)	15.9	10.9

What is Cholesterol?

Steroids are a group of compounds that contain seventeen carbon atoms arranged three 6-carbon rings and one 5-carbon ring. Sterols have a hydroxyl group (-OH) attached to the first 6-carbon ring.

Cholesterol is the main sterol in animal products, which is found in animal tissues, eggs, and dairy products. Cholesterol is a precursor of hormones (for example, testosterone, estrogen, progesterone, and cortisol), bile acids, and vitamin D. Sterols are found in plants (β-sitosterol, campesterol, and stigmasterol) and fungi (ergosterol). Ergosterol is a component of fungal cell membranes.

Cholesterol is a component of cell membranes and serves to make the cell membrane more rigid. Plants have cell walls comprising of polysaccharides (cellulose, hemicellulose, and pectin), which provides the rigidity.

Cholesterol is a waxy substance that is insoluble in water. It is transported in the blood by lipoproteins. There are five classes of lipoproteins, which are based on their size. Chylomicrons are the largest. Note that the intermediate density lipoproteins does not lie between the low and the high density lipoproteins.[94]

Lipoprotein	Origin	Composition (%)	Functions
Chylomicrons	Intestine	Triglycerides: 80-90 Cholesterol: 2-7 Phospholipids: 3-9	Transport of dietary triglycerides, originate in intestine
Very low density lipoprotein	Liver	Triglycerides: 55-80 Cholesterol: 5-15 Phospholipids: 10-20	Transport of synthesized triglycerides, originate in liver
Intermediate density lipoprotein	Metabolism of VLDL	Triglycerides: 20-50 Cholesterol: 20-40 Phospholipids: 15-25	Transport of cholesterol, originate via the metabolism of VLDL
Low density lipoprotein	Metabolism of VLDL and IDL	Triglycerides: 5-15 Cholesterol: 40-50 Phospholipids: 10-14	Transport of cholesterol, originate via the metabolism of VLDL and IDL
High density lipoprotein	Liver, intestine, intravascular metabolic reactions	Triglycerides: 5-10 Cholesterol: 15-25 Phospholipids: 20-30	Facilitates the removal of cholesterol, originate in intestine, liver

What is Heart Disease?

Endothelial cells line all blood (arteries, veins, capillaries as well as the heart) and lymphatic vessels. The endothelium is one cell thick.[95]

- When we eat a high-fat (or even a medium fat) standard Western diet, it increases the viscosity of the blood. White and red blood cells, platelets, endothelial cells, and low-density lipoprotein (LDL) particles containing cholesterol become adhesive— our blood becomes "sticky".
- The LDL particles, which contain cholesterol, enter into the space beneath the endothelium.
- The cholesterol becomes oxidized by free radicals. The activity of free radicals is greatly increased by eating oil, dairy, and animal protein.
- Macrophages cross into the sub-endothelial space and engulf LDL particles containing oxidized cholesterol. Macrophages are a type of white blood cell (or leukocyte), which are components of the immune system. Macrophages are comparatively long-lived white blood cells. After they have engulfed the offending intruder, information regarding the invader is passed to T-cells so it is easier for the immune system to deal with similar invaders in the future.
- After the macrophage engulfs its share of LDL particles, it dies. A macrophage that has engulfed LDL particles is known as a foam cell. Nikolaj

Anitschkow described and beautifully illustrated foam cells in the early 1900s.

- Plaques develop in the sub-endothelial space. Plaques consist of macrophages, foam cells, dead foam cells, fats, cholesterol, and smooth muscle tissue. The plaques intrude into the arteries.
- Thrombosis (blood clot inside a blood vessel) at the site of a ruptured plaque precipitates most heart attacks (myocardial infarctions).
- The vessel may become completely blocked. If this is a small blood vessel within the brain, the person may not be aware of the situation. If it is a large vessel, the person will have a heart attack or a stroke.

• • • • •

The endothelial cells produce nitric oxide. Nitric oxide dilates blood vessels and it also prevents cells in your blood from becoming adhesive.

Nitroglycerine is used to treat vascular conditions as it produces nitric oxide in the body.

A number of steps are involved in the production of nitric oxide, which can be blocked at different stages.[96]

- L-arginine is an amino acid that is relatively high in plant foods such as beans, legumes, nuts, fruit, and vegetables.

- Asymmetric dimethyl arginine (ADMA) interferes with the production of nitric oxide—too much ADMA then the production of nitric oxide falls.
- Dimethyl arginine dimethyl amino hydrolase (DDAH) destroys ADMA.

A number of factors prevent endothelial cells from producing nitric oxide by destroying the ability of DDAH to destroy ADMA. These include:

- hypertension (high blood pressure)
- high cholesterol
- high homocysteine
- high triglycerides, which includes all oils and fats including "healthy" oils
- insulin resistance, which is caused by high fat content in muscle cells
- smoking

If you have a high-fat meal then it compromises your ability to produce nitric oxide and at takes several hours to recover—just in time for your next high-fat meal.[97]

Healthy endothelial cells are essential to our health so doing everything possible to keep them from being damaged is imperative for our well-being.

• • • • •

Keeping our blood vessels healthy is a key to many diseases and conditions.

Our kidneys are rich in fine blood vessels. Kidneys are involved with filtering of the blood, absorption of nutrients, blood pressure regulation, and maintaining correct pH levels of blood.

We can limit our risk of heart disease and other "diseases of affluence" by taking a number of steps. Addressing only one issue, such as taking a tablet to reduce cholesterol, does not address other factors that are essential for optimal health.

• • • • •

Some dietary changes that diminish the amount of cholesterol in the blood are: reducing saturated fats consumption; reducing animal protein consumption; and reducing cholesterol consumption.

Colorful fruit, beans, and vegetables have high level of vitamins, minerals, and phytochemicals act as anti-oxidants, which assist in preventing the inflammation stage.

Homocysteine is a non-protein amino acid. It is synthesized in the body from methionine, which is a sulfur containing amino-acid. Methionine is much more prevalent in animal products than plant products. Rotten eggs smell the way they do because the sulfur produces a number of sulfur containing gasses including hydrogen sulfide—rotten egg gas.

A high level is of homocysteine is associated with an increased risk for chronic inflammation, cardiovascular disease, and Alzheimer's disease.

High levels may indicate vitamin B12, B6, or folic acid (B9) deficiency. It can also be caused by smoking, alcoholism, hypothyroidism, kidney disease, and diabetes. There are also genetic conditions that result in high homocysteine levels.

Optimal level of homocysteine is 6 µmol/L or lower. This may be lower than the reference range given by your pathology laboratory.

During the time of human evolution, the amount of omega-6 fatty acids in the food supply has increased and omega-3 fatty acids has decreased, from an estimated ratio of approximately 1:1 to 10:1–25:1, based on various estimates. Omega-3 fatty acids decrease platelet aggregation, blood viscosity, and fibrinogen production (involved in blood clot formation).[98]

Decreasing the amount of omega-6 oils (found in grains, corn, safflower, sunflower and cottonseed) is a better way of decreasing the omega-6 to omega-3 ratio than increasing the amount of omega-3 rich foods such as fish, fish oil and flaxseed oil.

To ensure an adequate amount of omega-3 oil in the diet, grind 20ml (1 tablespoon) of flaxseed in a spice grinder and add to meals each day. In order to be digested, the flaxseed needs to be ground. It is best to grind the flaxseed each day to prevent the oils from becoming oxidized.

5

A Very Brief History of Cardiovascular Research

Nikolaj Anitschkow – Atherosclerotic lesions in rabbits

It is convenient to place the origins of cardiovascular research to the second decade of the twentieth century.

In 1913, a 28-year-old pathologist, Nikolaj Anitschkow, working at the Military Medical Academy in St. Petersburg, showed that by feeding rabbits cholesterol dissolved in sunflower oil induced vascular lesions closely resembling those of human atherosclerosis. Controls fed only the sunflower oil showed no lesions.[99]

Steiner and Kendall – Atherosclerotic lesions in dogs

In 1946, Steiner and Kendall showed that by inhibiting the thyroid function in dogs and then feeding them cholesterol increases blood cholesterol and induces lesions. Under normal conditions, rats, dogs, and other carnivores are efficient at converting excess cholesterol to bile acids. It is impossible to produce atherosclerosis in dogs by feeding them a high-fat diet, without inhibiting their thyroid function.

John Gofman – Lipoproteins and their transport functions

By the 1950s, a number of important advances had been made including the discovery of the mechanism for cholesterol transportation in the blood (via lipoproteins) and the mechanism for cholesterol to enter the artery wall from the blood. Dr John Gofman was a leading pioneer researcher in the field of lipoproteins who was familiar with Anitschkow's work. His work showed that cholesterol and low-density lipoproteins were both indicators of coronary heart disease risk. This work and other evidence convinced Gofman that blood cholesterol, and the dietary determinants of blood cholesterol were centrally important in atherosclerosis. His wife, Dr Helen F Gofman co-authored a low-fat, low-cholesterol diet book[100] that was published in 1951. John Gofman wrote the preface for the book.

Ancel Keys

Authors such as: Uffe Ravnskov (*The Cholesterol Myths* – 1991); Gary Taubes (*Why We are Fat* – 2011, *Good Calories, Bad Calories* – 2007); Robert Lustig (*Fat Chance: Beating the Odds against Sugar, Processed Food, Obesity, and Disease* – 2013); and John Yudkin (*Pure, White and Deadly* – 1972) argue that cholesterol is *not* a health issue and concentrate on carbohydrates in the diet.

One method of advocating their case is to dismiss the work of Ancel Keys. Low-carbohydrate advocates claim he deliberately misled generations of researchers, medical practitioners, and the general public by manipulating data to fit his hypothesis.

A brief biography of Ancel Keys can be found in *Dialogues in Cardiovascular Medicine* that gives a different picture from the deceptive and manipulative researcher than he is portrayed by populist commentators. Below is a brief overview of his life.

• • • • •

Ancel Keys was one of the most influential public health researchers of the twentieth century. He was born in 1904 and died in 2004. He traveled extensively throughout his life. He was born in Colorado before moving to California at a young age. He attended University of California, studying economics, political science, and zoology. He obtained a Ph.D. in oceanography and biology before attaining his second Ph.D. at Cambridge in physiology. He married Margaret Haney in 1939—the same year, he was appointed professor of physiology at the University of Minnesota.[101]

During World War II, he instigated an experiment to determine the effects of starvation on 36 conscientious objectors. This helped to develop programs to assist the rehabilitation of those who had been starved during the war. The men "universally stated a simple, solid conviction not to kill another human being," of their dedication to the experiment, and their desire to be of service to those who were starving in appalling conditions in Europe. Keys was remembered for his professionalism and compassion. It is a reflection of Keys and his staff that the participants insisted that they would "make the same decision to participate, even after having experienced the physical sacrifice required."[102]

Keys demonstrated that traits such as body type, blood fat levels, cholesterol, blood pressure, heart rate, and responses to stress were able to be changed—attributes that were considered to be innate.[103]

In 1951, Keys was working at Oxford when the Food and Agriculture Organization asked him to chair their first conference on nutrition in Rome. He states, "The conferees talked only about nutritional deficiencies". When he asked about the new epidemic of coronary heart disease, Gino Bergami, Professor of Physiology at the University of Naples, said "coronary heart disease was no problem in Naples".

In 1952, Keys and his wife Margaret visited Naples. Margaret measured serum cholesterol concentrations and found them to be very low except among members of the Rotary Club. Heart attacks were rare except amongst the rich whose diet included daily servings of meat. He obtained similar results in studies in Madrid.

In Minnesota, he performed a series of experiments that lasted for eight years with the results published in 1965. According to Keys:

The major villains in the diet that are responsible for raising the concentration of cholesterol in the blood serum are saturated fatty acids in the fat of meat and dairy products. Preformed cholesterol in the diet also tends to raise blood cholesterol concentrations slightly if the diet otherwise is extremely low in cholesterol. Mark Hegsted at Harvard University confirmed our Minnesota findings in similar experiments. Saturated fatty acids and preformed cholesterol are commonly found in the same foods. The good Mediterranean diet is low in both saturated fat and cholesterol.[104]

Keys stressed on a number of occasions that there were "differences in population versus individual causes of heart disease."

When groups of individuals are compared, all measurements invariably show statistically significant correlations between the measurements and the presence or absence of the tendency towards heart disease. But the correlations are far from perfect and the reliability is low for single individuals.[105]

Ancel Keys coined the name and introduced the concept of Mediterranean diet. In 1975, Ancel Keys and his wife Margaret published the book, *How to Eat Well and Stay Well the Mediterranean Way*,[106] based on the results of his studies.

Ancel Keys and his wife Margaret lived for 28 years in Pioppi, a fishing village south of Naples in southern Italy. Keys lived to be 100 years old and his wife 97. Margaret was a biochemist and was an integral part of Keys's work.

Goldstein and Brown – Discovery of the LDL Receptor

Joseph Goldstein and Michael Brown[107] met at Massachusetts General Hospital in Boston after completing their medical degrees in 1966. After completing their internships, they obtained research positions at the National Institutes of Health in Bethesda, Maryland. As well as performing separate research, they both attended their clinical patients.

Joseph Goldstein encountered patients with familial hypercholesterolemia (FH). This condition is caused by a single gene, a monogenic condition. This can result in serum cholesterol levels of up to 25 mmol/L (1,000 mg/dL) and result in deposits of cholesterol and fats in places on the body such as around the eyelids and tendons. Atherosclerosis and subsequent heart attacks may occur in the first decade of life.

Goldstein and Brown[108] merged their laboratories in 1972 at the University of Texas Southwestern Medical Center in Dallas. They discovered the low-density lipoprotein (LDL) receptors on the surface of cells that bind to the low-density lipoproteins (LDL) that transport cholesterol. This allows cholesterol to enter the cells from the blood. FH patients lack sufficient LDL receptors, resulting in cholesterol-related diseases. This work earned them the Nobel Prize in Physiology or Medicine in 1985.

Brown and Goldstein's discovery of scavenger receptors on macrophage (a type of white blood cell that engulfs foreign particles) cells[109] was another of their important findings. Macrophages cross into the sub-endothelial space and engulf the LDL that contain oxidized cholesterol. The process of inflammation was (and still is by some popular commentators) regarded as a competing hypothesis to the role of fats and cholesterol in heart disease. However, the inflammatory process is always preceded by high serum cholesterol.

In a speech at the 2006 International Achievement Summit in Los Angeles, Brown tells the Academy's students that heart disease is totally preventable.

> The good news is that it [heart disease] is total preventable. We do not need a vaccine, we do not need a new discovery, we do not even need stem cells. We know how to prevent heart disease and heart attacks right now.
>
> The problem has been switched from one of science to one of social policy and human behavior. And it turns out to be a lot easier to do the science than to change people's behavior.
>
> The real news is that we shouldn't really need these drugs [statins]. That for those of us who have normal genes, the reason why our blood is

being filled up with cholesterol is because we are basically eating too much cholesterol and too much animal fat. And if you look at populations where the diet is lower in cholesterol and fat, they don't need these statin drugs, they have low cholesterols in their blood, and they have twenty times lower rate of heart attacks than we do in the United States.

Cholesterol skeptics ignore the extensive work of Goldstein and Brown and do not attempt to dispute their results.

6

Review of Important Studies

Framingham Heart Study

Framingham is located in eastern Massachusetts, 30 km west of Boston with a current population of 70,000 people.

The Framingham Heart Study[110] began in 1948. The population of Framingham at that time was about 28,000 people. The purpose was to examine factors that influence cardiovascular health. This was a joint project of the National Heart, Lung, and Blood Institute and Boston University with the objective to identify the causes of heart disease and stroke—the largest (and growing) cause of death in the U.S. 5,209 people between the ages of 30–62 with no apparent symptoms of heart disease were involved.

Since 1948, the subjects have continued to return to the study every two years for a detailed follow-up reviews. The second generation of participants were enrolled in 1971, resulting in 5,124 of the original participants' adult children and their spouses participating. Since 2002, a third generation of participants have been involved.

This study lead to the identification of the major heart disease risk factors: high blood pressure, high blood cholesterol, smoking, obesity, diabetes, and physical inactivity.

Evaluation of the 10-year follow up identified higher cholesterol, higher blood pressure and smoking as the major risks. The term *Risk Factor* for heart disease originated within this study. If one factor was abnormal the risk doubled— two abnormal factors increased the risk 3.5 times—all three abnormal, the risk increased 10 times.

Blood pressure of greater than or equal to 130/85 mmHg is considered high. The risk increases when cholesterol is equal to or greater than 4.4 mmol/L (170 mg/dL). The higher the cholesterol over this value the higher the risk.[111] For most practitioners, cholesterol levels of less than 5.2 mmol/L (200 mg/dL) are usually considered desirable.

Lester Morrison's Diet-Heart Study

Lester Morrison was a cardiologist located in Los Angeles, California. He was aware of the experiments of Nikolaj Anitschkow, which appears to be unusual for the time.

Morrison wrote in 1955 that:

> The incrimination of dietary fat as the cause of human arteriosclerosis or atherosclerosis dates largely from World War I. After the British blockade of Germany during that war, it was noted extensively by German pathologists and

clinicians that the incidence of deaths and sickness from coronary and cerebral vascular atherosclerosis fell sharply.[112]

He decided as early as 1946 that lowering blood cholesterol might be therapeutic and began possibly the first study testing the possible benefit of cholesterol lowering. His study consisted of one hundred people, mostly men. Every second person was assigned to a low-fat, low-cholesterol diet. The others were told to maintain their usual diet. The total daily fat intake in this diet was 25 g with animal fats eaten in minimum quantities.

By the end of twelve years, nine of the fifty patients treated with the diet survived. All of the fifty control patients had died by the twelfth year. The experimental group's cholesterol fell from 312 mg/dl to 220 mg/dl (8.1 mmol/L to 5.7 mmol/L)—a 30% decrease.[113]

Currently, a cholesterol level of 5.7 mmol/L is not considered to be low.

Morrison also advocated the use of lecithin and choline to reduce cholesterol and repair damage to arterial walls. He wrote 150 scientific papers and 2 books—*The Low Fat Way to Health and Longer Life* and *Dr Morrison's Heart-Saver Program.*

Ancel Keys's Atherosclerosis: A Problem in Newer Public Health paper

Popular commentators frequently accuse Keys of manipulating data in his 1953 paper, *Atherosclerosis, A Problem in Newer Public Health*. This study is sometimes referred as the "Six Countries Study". A number of popular commentators think this is the *Seven Countries Study*—they count *England & Wales* as two countries.

This paper was presented in Amsterdam in 1952 and in January 1953 in New York.

On page 4 of this paper, Keys lists 16 countries (which includes France, Switzerland, and Sweden) and compared their all-cause death rates to the United States. United States compared unfavorably to most countries and Keys believed that what was possible for other countries "should be possible for Americans." The mortality data was for the years 1947–1949.

On page 17 of this 22-page paper, Keys graphed the mortality rate for degenerative heart disease and fat intake for six countries that he stated had "fully comparable dietary and vital statistics data." The food data was obtained from FAO for the year 1949.

This graph causes a great deal of consternation in the popular press. The claim is made that Keys "cherry-picked" his data, which is stating that he was dishonest.

Yerushalmy and Hilleboe criticized this paper in the publication *Fat in the Diet and Mortality from Heart Disease*,[114] claiming that Keys only choose 6 countries (Japan, Italy, England & Wales, Australia, Canada, U.S.) that supported his hypothesis instead of using the World Health Organization data from the 22 countries that was available. The data for the 22 countries that Yerushalmy and Hilleboe listed were for the years 1951-1953, a period which is after the publication of Keys's paper.

Even if data from *all the 22 countries* are included, it still shows:

- positive correlations between heart disease and total calories consumed, fat consumption, animal fat consumption, and animal protein consumption, and
- negative correlations with heart disease and carbohydrate consumption, vegetable protein consumption, and vegetable fat consumption.

This observation is clearly stated in Yerushalmy and Hilleboe's paper. They were disputing the methodology—not the absence of correlation. The paper also states that Keys did not give reasons for his selection. This is incorrect. Keys did give the reasons for choices.

The Scandinavian countries were excluded because of the effects of the World War II. The consumption of meat and eggs dropped during the war and so did the level of heart disease. A graph from a paper published in 1951 shows a dramatic decrease in deaths rates shortly after the Nazi invasion of Norway. Age-adjusted mortality from circulatory diseases in Norway rose from 27 per 10,000 to 35 per 10,000 during the years 1927–1939, prior to the outbreak of World War II. By 1945, the rate had dropped 30% to 24 per 10,000 and immediately started rising in the year that followed.[115]

It was known at the time that France had a different methodology for categorizing heart disease than other countries. The WHO data shows France as having little heart disease even though it has a high fat consumption, giving rise to the French Paradox myth. According to a paper in *The Dialogues of Medicine*, the French Paradox is indeed a myth:

> The clear conclusion, driven by the facts as summarized by Pierre Ducimetière, is that the rates of CHD are not so low in France, animal fat intake is not so high, and the diet-heart concept is not so unique that the existence of a "French paradox" can be sustained, except for satisfying cultural fantasy or for wine enthusiasm and marketing. Thus, the real paradox is why the French paradox continues to exist as a concept, when it should be replaced by the less mystifying view, namely, "the more Mediterranean, the better".[116]

Spain was excluded even though these figures supported the conclusions of the paper. Mexico did not have a death certificate system in place.

Hilleboe later co-authored a paper *Risk Factors in Ischemic Heart Disease.* The study divided the population into three groups based on cholesterol levels: low, medium, and high. The paper stated, "The nearly threefold difference in rate [for the incidence of heart disease] for the high level cholesterol group over the low is the greatest for any single variable."[117]

Yerushalmy was later involved in a disagreement with researchers who claimed that women who smoked had lower birth-weight infants. He suggested that smoking was not the cause of the lower birth weight but a result of "mode of life" differences between the smoking population and non-smoking population.

• • • • •

In 1959, Norman Jolliffe and Morton Archer published a paper, *Statistical associations between international coronary heart disease death rates and certain environmental factors,*[118] that examined Yerushalmy and Hilleboe's conclusions. Jolliffe and Archer state that Yerushalmy and Hilleboe erred in disregarding the distinction between saturated fat and polyunsaturated fat, in relation to heart disease. This distinction was not known when Keys wrote his original paper.

Joliffe and Archer state that "the intake of saturated types of fat was most important in accounting for the differences in coronary heart disease death rates. Of somewhat lesser importance, the intake of animal protein also accounted for a large proportion of the explained variance in these death rates."

Norman Jolliffe published data for death rates of B-26 category of deaths. B-26 category referred to *Arteriosclerotic and degenerative heart disease.* Jolliffe used data for 20 countries from *World Health Organization: Annual Epidemiological and Vital Statistics* for the year 1955.

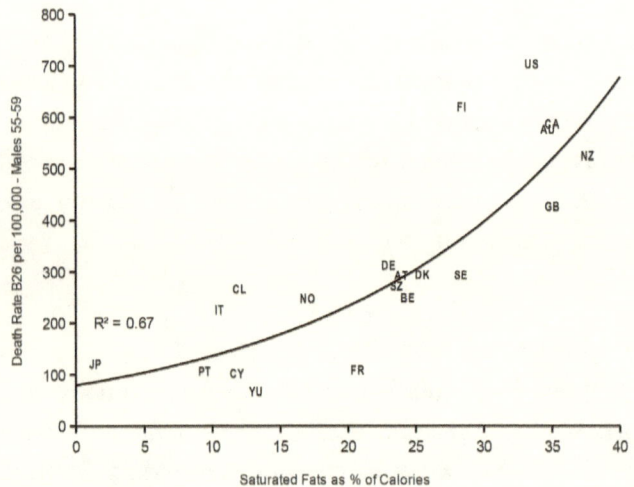

AT Austria; AU Australia; BE Belgium; CA Canada; CL Chile; CY Ceylon; DE Germany; DK Denmark; FI Finland; FR France; GB United Kingdom; IT Italy; JP Japan; NO Norway; NZ New Zealand; PT Portugal; SE Sweden; SZ Switzerland; US United States; YU Yugoslavia

The graph shows an exponential correlation between the death rate and saturated fat consumption. The coefficient of determination (R^2) is 0.67, which is a significant correlation. A similar correlation ($R^2 = 0.66$) exists with the death rate and animal protein consumption.[119]

• • • • •

Critics commonly mistake the *"Six Countries Study"* with the later *Seven Countries Study* published in 1970. They also state that this was a very influential paper. Teicholz claims that this paper received "enormous attention" and that "this connect-the-dot exercise in 1952 was the acorn that grew into the giant oak tree of our mistrust of fat today". This assertion does not appear to be true. Keys stated, after the initial presentation in Amsterdam in 1952, that "few among the large audience accepted my thesis of an important association between the diet and the incidence of coronary heart disease." It is a minor discussion paper.

In recent years, far too much attention is paid to one page of a discussion paper written in the early 1950s. Keys writes, "The fact that the present high rate from degenerative heart disease in the United States is not inevitable is easily shown by the comparison with some other countries." This was the purpose of the paper.

The Wadsworth Veterans Administration Hospital Study, 1969

The Wadsworth VA Hospital in Los Angeles operated a home where male army veterans resided. The meals were provided by one of two dining halls.[120]

Men in dining hall A continued their usual diet. The "saturated animal fat and hydrogenated shortening replaced with vegetable oils in the experimental diet" for the diets provided in dining hall B. Low-fat diets were not considered because such a diet required "gastronomic sacrifice." The total fat content of the two diets were the same, providing 40% of the total energy. Diets of 40% fat cannot be considered a healthy diet.

Both groups were told that their diet had changed. Compliance rates 56% for the control diet and 49% for experimental diet.

846 men, most of them in their 60s or 70s, were randomly assigned to one or the other dining room and followed for up to 8 years. Average age at the start of the study was 65.5. The study was carried out in the late 1950s by Seymour Dayton and Morton Pearce from the University of California.

The blood cholesterol of the experimental group fell 12.7%. The number of events (definite heart attack, fatal or nonfatal; stroke; or peripheral atherosclerosis requiring amputation) was reduced by 31% in the experimental group (48 versus 70).[121]

This is how David Gillespie commented on the trial in *Toxic Oil*:

> A much larger trial, completed in 1971, was conducted with a population of 846 Californian military veterans in domiciled care randomly assigned to two different diets. In the Veterans Trial, one kitchen replaced all animal-fat products with corn oil for the eight-year duration of the study. The other kitchen kept on serving a normal high-animal-fat diet. As expected, the corn-oil group had a lower average blood-cholesterol

level by the end of the trial, although the 'improvement' (13 per cent) wasn't as great as in the London Hospital Study. Heart-disease-related events were slightly fewer than expected in both groups, but not significantly different from each other. But what really concerned the researchers was the dramatic difference in cancer deaths between the two groups. The incidence of fatal cancers in the corn-oil group was nearly double that of the normal-diet group.[122]

Gillespie transforms the significant 31% reduction in cardiovascular events to be "not significantly different from each other". Similarly, he transforms the non-significant increase in carcinoma deaths into a finding that "really concerned the researchers".

Seymour Dayton reported his findings in *The Lancet*:

Many of the cancer deaths in the experimental group were among those who did not adhere closely to the diet. This reduces the possibility that the feeding of polyunsaturated oils was responsible for the excess carcinoma mortality observed in the experimental group. [...]

During the late part of the trial there was a crossover of the curves for total death-rates due to an excess non-atherosclerotic mortality among experimental subjects. In this phase of the trial, numbers were relatively small and the excess non-atherosclerotic mortality after the sixth anniversary accounted for 9 cases. The differences in non-atherosclerotic deaths in this period was entirely due to trauma (0 controls, 4 experimental) and to carcinoma (2 controls, 7 experimental).

The author does point out that these differences occurred only in the older group of veterans—not in the younger group. There is also a difference in smoking patterns between the experimental and control groups. The authors state that "this is probably not significant". The paper states that the difference in cancer rates between the two groups is "non-significant". This is far from a finding that "really concerned the researchers."

MJ Karvonen from Finland reported on diets high in polyunsaturated fats and incidence of cancer:

In the Los Angeles veterans study, a statistically non-significant excess of cancer incidence and of cancer mortality was reported among those on the experimental diet (Dayton et al. 1969; Pearce & Dayton, 1971). This, however, has not been the rule in other similar studies. And when the results of five studies (Oslo, London, Helsinki, Faribault and Los Angeles) were combined, the total mortality of those on the diet was only 85% of that of their controls. There was no significant difference in cancer incidence or mortality in the combined material.[123]

The premise that diets high in polyunsaturated fats contribute to cancer cannot be substantiated.

Ancel Keys's Seven Countries Study

Ancel Keys and colleagues posed the hypothesis that differences among populations in the frequency of heart attacks and stroke would occur as a result of physical characteristics and lifestyle and diet.

Surveys were carried out between 1958-1970 in populations of men aged 40-59, in sixteen areas of seven countries. Follow-up surveys were continued until the 1990s. A total of 12,763 men were enrolled in the program.

Preliminary studies were carried out in Italy and the Greek island of Crete in 1957. A preliminary study was also performed in Hawaii. American men of European background were compared with Japanese living in Japan and Hawaii. The Japanese, who consumed a traditional Japanese diet had cholesterol levels of 4.1 mmol/L (160 mg/dL) whilst Americans in Hawaii had similar cholesterol to those on the mainland.

Most of the areas were stable and rural and had wide contrasts in their normal diet. Women were excluded because cardiac disease in women was much less common and because of the invasiveness of physical examinations.

The *Seven Countries Study* was the first to explore associations among diet, risk, and disease in contrasting populations. A centralized chemical analysis of foods consumed among randomly selected families in each area and a diet-recall for all the men, allowed an effective test of the dietary hypothesis. The study was unique for its time, in standardization of measurements of diet, risk factors, and disease; training its survey teams; and central, blindfold coding and analysis of data.

The study areas were: one area is in the United States, two areas in Finland, one area in the Netherlands, three areas in Italy, five areas in the former Yugoslavia (two in Croatia, and three in Serbia), two areas in Greece (Crete, Corfu), and two areas in Japan.

Teicholz claims, "A number of critics have since pointed out that had Keys taken the critiques of Yerushalmy to heart, he might have selected a European country to challenge his fat hypothesis, like Switzerland or France (or Germany or Norway or Sweden). Instead, he chose only those nations (based on national statistics) that seemed likely to confirm it."

Jolliffe (1959),[124] using data from 20 countries, showed a strong correlation with saturated fat and heart disease. This data included Switzerland, France, Germany, Norway, and Sweden.

Artaud-Wild et al (1993),[125] using data from 40 countries, showed a strong correlation with the Cholesterol-Saturated Fat Index per 1000 kcal/day. Even though Artaud-Wild is the lead author of this paper, it is known as the Connor study.

France and Finland were outliers in both studies—Finland having a higher than expected death rate and France a lower rate. The conclusion of the Connor study is "the country in which people also consume more plant foods, including small amounts of liquid vegetable oils, and more vegetables (more antioxidants) had lower rates of CHD mortality. On the other hand, milk and butterfat were associated with increased CHD mortality." French people also consume less food than the Finns.

The Connor study also examined the relationship with heart disease and milk intake—the milk intake was measured per 1000 kcal/day, not the total intake—and heart disease. It showed a similar correlation but France and Finland were no longer outliers.

There are strong regional variations in diet and disease patterns in France. A north-south-east gradient exists for all-cause mortality, cardiovascular mortality, hypertension, obesity, and high lipids.[126] A study involving French women born between 1925 and 1950 showed that the north has a greater consumption of: fat products, butter, margarine, potatoes, processed meat, alcohol, coffee, and saturated fats; and has a lower consumption of fiber than the rest of France.[127] There is also a higher prevalence of multiple sclerosis in the north-east and a lower prevalence in Paris and the Mediterranean.[128]

• • • • •

A number of other variables were recorded along with fat and saturated fat intake:

- demographic factors including occupation
- smoking, physical activity and dietary pattern
- medical history
- height, weight, skinfold measurements, mid-arm circumference
- blood pressure
- heart and lung auscultation, peripheral pulses, fundus examination
- electrocardiogram and resting heart rate
- biochemical tests including serum lipids. The lipoprotein fractions and serum uric acid tests were not included because of financial constraints.
- respiratory function measurements

Follow-up examination surveys after five and ten years were part of the initial plan and were performed in all regions except for the 5-year examination in Japan and the 10-year examination of the U.S. railroad personnel.

Ancel Keys wrote *Seven Countries: A Multivariate Analysis of Death and Coronary Heart Disease* (1980), a 380-page book, which documented the results of the 10-year follow-up.[129]

There was a significant correlation between the 10-year incidence of coronary deaths and the percentage of saturated fat in the diet (r = 0.84). The relationship between the 10-year incidence of coronary deaths and the percentage of total fat in the diet is not nearly as significant (r = 0.50).

Note the Keys used the word *partly* in his overview of the conclusions following the ten-year follow-up:

The differences found in the Seven Countries Study were partly explained by differences in the blood pressure, serum cholesterol, and the typical diets of the cohorts.[130]

Cardiovascular risk factors were also examined by repeat surveys in nine European regions after 25, 30, 35, and 40 years follow-up.

The *Seven Countries Study* provided evidence: for the concept of sick and healthy populations; that the major cardiovascular risk factors are universal; for the diet-heart hypothesis; that cardiovascular disease is preventable; and that a healthy lifestyle may promote different aspects of health.

Seventh-day Adventist's Studies

A strong commitment to health has been a part of Adventist's tradition since its founding in the 1840s.

There has been three large Adventist cohort studies in the United States and Canada. These studies have generated hundreds of papers, which give a valuable insight to diet and the implication for our health.[131]

- Adventist Mortality Study (1960-1976)   22,940 participants
- Adventist Health Study – 1 (1976 – 1980)   34,198 participants
- Adventist Health Study – 2 (Started 2002)   96,194 participants

Data from the AHS-2 study shows that Adventists smoke much less frequently than the general American population (males - 1.2%, females – 1.0%) and drink less alcohol (6.6% drink alcohol).

Diet is also significantly different from the general population with 4.2% being total vegetarian, 31.6% lacto-ovo-vegetarian, 11.4% include fish with their lacto-ovo-vegetarian diet, 6.1% semi-vegetarian (eat meat <1 time/week) and 46.8% non-vegetarian.

• • • • •

The AHS-1 study showed 30-year-old Adventist males lives 7.3 years longer than the average 30-year-old white Californian male and with females living 4.4 years longer than the average Californian white female. For vegetarians, it is 9.5 years longer for men and 6.1 years longer for women.

This study also shows that early menarche was associated with increased total mortality, ischemic heart disease and stroke. A one-year delay in menarche was associated with 4.5% lower total mortality.[132]

AHS-1 showed that women who consumed tomatoes three or four times a week reduced the rate of ovarian cancer by 70%. Tomato consumption is also related to a decrease in prostate cancer in men. Adventists, who ate meat, had a 65% increased risk of colon cancer compared to the vegetarian Adventists. Men drinking five to six glasses of water a day had a 60-70% reduction of the incidence of a fatal heart attack.[133]

• • • • •

The comparison of the types of diet (in the AHS-2) showed a significant difference in both the body weight and the incidence of Type 2 Diabetes.[134]

Category	%	BMI (kg / m^2)	Prevalence Type 2 Diabetes (%)	Odd ratio (*)
Vegan No red meat, fish, poultry, dairy, eggs	4.2	23.6	2.9	0.51
Lacto-ovo vegetarians Vegan with eggs and milk	31.6	25.7	3.2	0.54
Pesco-vegetarians Vegan with fish, milk and eggs	11.4	26.3	4.8	0.70
Semi-vegetarians Red meat, poultry less than once a week plus fish, milk, and eggs	6.1	27.3	6.1	0.76
Non-vegetarians Red meat, poultry, fish, milk and eggs more than once a week	46.8	28.8	7.6	1

(*) **After adjustment for age, sex, ethnicity, education, income, physical activity, television watching, sleep habits, alcohol use and BMI.**

The differences in outcomes depending upon diet type are listed below. Lacto-ovo-vegetarian and vegan outcomes are compared with non-vegetarian outcomes.

Cardio-metabolic factors	Lacto-ovo-vegetarian	Vegan
Hypertension	0.45	0.25
Diabetes	0.39	0.22
Type-2 diabetes	0.54	0.51
Diabetes mellitus	0.62	0.38

Relative Risk or Odds Ratio of cardio-metabolic-related factors among vegan and lacto-ovo-vegetarian Adventists compared with non-vegetarians

Cancer-specific site	Lacto-ovo-vegetarian	Vegan
All cancers	0.95	0.86
Gastrointestinal	0.76	0.80
Respiratory tract	0.85	0.59
Urinary tract	1.13	1.73
All-male cancers	0.95	0.81
All-female cancers	1.04	0.71

Hazard ratio of all-cancer and site-specific cancers among vegan and lacto-ovo-vegetarian Adventists compared with non-vegetarians

Cause of Mortality	Lacto-ovo-vegetarian	Vegan
All-cause mortality	0.91	0.85
• Males	0.86	0.72
• Females	0.94	0.97
All-cancer	0.90	0.92
• Males	1.01	0.81
• Females	0.85	0.99
Ischemic heart disease	0.82	0.90
• Males	0.76	0.45
• Females	0.85	1.39
Cardiovascular disease	0.90	0.91
• Males	0.77	0.58

• Females	0.99	1.18
Other causes	0.91	0.74
• Males	0.89	0.81
• Females	0.93	0.70

Hazard ratio of all-cause and cause-specific mortality among lacto-ovo-vegetarians and vegan Adventists compared with non-vegetarians.

As the diet becomes more vegetarian then the risk factors decreased for all categories except for female ischemic heart disease and female urinary tract cancers. Note that the comparisons are within the Adventist community, which is significantly healthier than the general U.S. population.

Lyon Diet Heart Study

The *Catalyst* program, *Heart of the Matter,* states that the *Lyon Diet Heart Study* provides evidence that cholesterol is not implicated in heart disease.

The *Lyon Diet Heart Study* is a "randomized, single-blind secondary prevention trial aimed at testing whether a Mediterranean-type diet, compared with a prudent Western-type diet, may reduce recurrence after a first myocardial infarction."

The study consisted of 605 patients who had recovered from a myocardial infarction at a hospital in southern France.

The experimental group emphasized more bread, vegetables and green vegetables, more fish, less beef, lamb and pork replaced with poultry, no day without fruit, and butter and cream replaced with margarine high in α-linolenic acid (an omega-3 fatty acid).[135]

After 27 months, the control group had 16 cardiac deaths and 17 non-fatal events whilst the experimental group had 3 deaths and 5 events.

The final report of the *Lyon Diet Heart Study*[136], states that cholesterol is indeed implicated in heart disease. The report states, "The data confirm the impressive protective effect of the Mediterranean diet." The report concludes:

> The major traditional risk factors, such as high blood cholesterol and blood pressure, were shown to be independent and joint predictors of recurrence, indicating that the Mediterranean dietary pattern did not alter, at least qualitatively, the usual relationships between major risk factors and recurrence.

This report also states:

> For each increase of 1 mmol/L of total cholesterol increased the risk of recurrence by 20% to 30%. Epidemiological studies have consistently shown a positive correlation between plasma cholesterol levels and the incidence of (and mortality from) CHD in various populations. Thus, our population does not appear to be different from other low-risk populations.

Multiple Risk Factor Intervention Trial (MRFIT)

The *Multiple Risk Factor Intervention Trial* (MRFIT) was a coronary heart disease prevention trial that was conducted at 22 U.S. clinical centers, in 18 cities, from 1973 to 1982. The multiple risks that were evaluated were: elevated serum cholesterol; elevated blood pressure; and cigarette smoking.

A number of popular commentators use this trial as proof that cholesterol is not implicated in heart disease. The tobacco industry also used the results of the MRFIT study to argue that smoking is not harmful.

12,866 men between the ages of 35-57 with one or more of these risk factors were randomly assigned to the "Special Intervention" (SI) or "Usual Care" (UC) group and followed for 6-8 years.

UC men were given information on risk factors, referred to their usual sources of care, and re-examined annually.

SI participants received group and individual counselling on a fat-modified diet, a drug-treatment program for diastolic hypertension (after an initial attempt at blood pressure control by weight reduction), and counselling for cigarette smokers.[137]

The mean values at the start of the trial and the mean values for the two groups after six years of intervention are shown in the following table.

Criteria	Units	Baseline	UC group	SI Group
Diastolic blood pressure	mmHg	91.0	83.7	80.5
Smoking rate	%	59%	46%	32%
Cholesterol	mg/dL	240.0	232.5	227.9
Cholesterol	mmol/L	6.2	6.0	5.9
Mortality – All-cause	per 1000		40.4	41.2
Mortality – CHD	per 1000		19.3	17.9

The results are not spectacular. All-cause mortality was greater in the SI group—although both mortality rates were not statistically significant. The blood pressure and blood cholesterol for both groups is still high. After six years of intervention, more impressive results should be expected.

Note that the UC group was not a "No Treatment" group. Both groups were making changes that resulted in lowering their risk factors. Deaths from cardiac disease was declining in the U.S., Canada, and Australia but not in the United Kingdom.

Initially, the drug hydrochlorothiazide was used in the trial to lower blood pressure. However, this drug: raises cholesterol;[138] causes left ventricular hypertrophy; and increases mortality.[139] The use of this drug did distort results.

The results after 16 years are a little more impressive. After 16 years, those who had been in the SI group experienced cardiac deaths at a rate 11.4% lower than the UC group and a total mortality rate 5.7% lower.

• • • • •

There were 356 222 men aged 35 to 57 years, who were free of a history of hospitalization for myocardial infarction, that were initially screened by the MRFIT program in its recruitment program.

This provided researchers with a group that had standardized serum cholesterol measurements and 6-year mortality follow-up. For the entire group, aged 35 to 57 years at entry, the age-adjusted risks of CHD death in cholesterol quintiles are shown below.[140]

Quintile	Cholesterol (mg/dL)	Cholesterol (mmol/L)	Age-Adjusted Risk
1	< 182	< 4.71	1
2	182 - 202	4.71 - 5.22	1.29
3	203 - 220	5.25 - 5.69	1.73
4	221 - 244	5.72 - 6.31	2.21
5	> 244	>6.31	3.42

The conclusion from this paper is:

> Data of high precision show that the relationship between serum cholesterol and CHD is not a threshold one, with increased risk confined to the two highest quintiles, but rather is a continuously graded one that powerfully affects risk for the great majority of middle-aged American men.

For these men that were initially screened for the MRFIT cohort and without a history of myocardial infarction, low risk was defined as: optimal level of serum cholesterol; optimal systolic and diastolic blood pressure; non-smoking; and no history of treatment for diabetes.

Only 2% of the men in the MRFIT cohort met these criteria. Only six of these men died from CHD during the 6-year follow-up, and the CHD death rate was 87% lower than for the rest of the cohort.[141]

Results from the MRFIT were used to determine the effects of polyunsaturated fatty acids on coronary heart disease.[142]

- No significant associations with mortality were detected for linolenic acid, the predominant dietary omega-6 fatty acid.
- Higher omega-3 fatty acid consumption resulted in lower death rates for coronary heart disease, all cardiovascular diseases, and all-cause mortality.
- Higher omega-3 to omega-6 ratio resulted in lower cancer mortality.

Women's Health Initiative

The *Women's Health Initiative* is a U.S. study involving 161,808 women aged 50-79. It investigated hormone therapy, dietary patterns, calcium, and vitamin D supplementation and their effects on the prevention of heart disease, cancer, and osteoporotic fractures.[143]

The study involved two major components: Clinical Trials; and an Observational Study.

The Clinical Trials studied three different aspects: a Hormone Therapy trial; a Dietary Modification trial; and a Calcium/Vitamin D trial.

The Observational Study examined the relationship between lifestyle, health and risk factors, and specific diseases outcomes. This component involves tracking the medical history and health habits of 93,676 women. Recruitment for this study was completed in 1998 and participants were followed for 8 to 12 years.

The Dietary Modification trial evaluated the effect of a low-fat and high-fruit, vegetable-and-grain diet on the prevention of breast and colorectal cancers, and coronary heart disease in post-menopausal women. The participants followed either their usual eating pattern or a low-fat dietary pattern.

The women were randomly assigned to the control group or intervention group. The women self-reported their diets. According to the study, the intervention consisted of:

> Intensive behavior modification in group and individual sessions designed to reduce total fat intake to 20% of calories and increase intakes of vegetables/fruits to 5 servings/d and grains to at least 6 servings/d. The comparison group received diet-related education materials.[144]

This was achieved by holding 18 group sessions in the first year and quarterly maintenance sessions afterwards for the intervention group. It could be disputed that this constitutes intensive behavior modification.

The widely-reported conclusion from this study informed readers that:

Over a mean of 8.1 years, a dietary intervention that reduced total fat intake and increased intakes of vegetables, fruits, and grains did not significantly reduce the risk of CHD, stroke, or CVD in postmenopausal women and achieved only modest effects on CVD risk.

Whilst the conclusion states that the mean period for the participants in the study was 8.1 years, the data shows changes at years 3 and 6.

	Baseline Mean		Year 3 Mean		Change at Year 3		
Risk factor	Int.	Comp.	Int.	Comp.	Int.	Comp.	Difference
Weight, kg	76.8	76.7	75.7	76.7	-0.7	0.6	-1.29
Body mass index	29.1	29.1	28.8	29.2	-0.2	0.3	-0.49
Waist circumference, cm	89.0	89.0	88.2	89.3	-0.4	0.5	-0.98
Blood pressure, mm Hg Systolic	127.5	127.9	125.1	125.7	-2.2	-2.1	-0.17
Cholesterol, mg/dL Total	224.0	224.2	214.1	216.6	-10.2	-6.9	-3.26

Differences between the Mean Changes in Cardiovascular Disease Risk Factors from Baseline to Year 3 in the Intervention Group and the Comparison Group

Dietary Intakes	Baseline		Change at Year 6		
	Int.	Comp.	Int.	Comp.	Difference
Total energy, kcal/d	1790.2	1789.4	1431.8	1546.2	-114.3
Total fat - % of energy	37.8	37.8	28.8	37.0	-8.2
Saturated fat - % of energy	12.7	12.7	9.5	12.4	-2.9
P/S fat ratio	0.6	0.6	0.7	0.6	0.0
Total trans fatty acid - % of energy	2.7	2.8	1.8	2.4	-0.6
Protein - % of energy	16.5	16.4	17.7	17.1	0.6
Carbohydrate - % of energy	45.6	45.6	53.9	45.9	8.1
Dietary fiber, g/day	15.4	15.4	16.9	14.4	2.4
Cholesterol, mg/day	260.5	260.0	193.6	243.5	-49.9

Dietary Intakes	Baseline		Change at Year 6		
	Int.	Comp.	Int.	Comp.	Difference
Vegetables and fruits - servings/day	3.6	3.6	4.9	3.8	1.1
Grains - servings/day	4.7	4.8	4.3	3.8	0.5
Whole grains - servings/day	1.1	1.1	1.2	1.0	0.2
Soy - servings/week	0.1	0.1	0.3	0.2	0.0
Nuts - servings/week	1.5	1.5	1.0	1.8	-0.8
Fish - servings/week	1.9	1.9	2.0	2.0	0.0

Mean Baseline and Follow-up Nutrient Intakes at 6 years

An examination of the tables reveals the following conclusions.

- There was very little change in both the control group and intervention group in the risk factors: body mass index; waist circumference; cholesterol; triglycerides; insulin resistance; and serum carotenoids. On average, the women were overweight at the start of the study and were overweight at the 3-year point, with an average weight loss of 1.29 kg. Their weight was not reported at the 6-year period.
- If the participants really did reduce the energy consumption by 20% then it would be expected that the weight loss would be much greater than indicated.
- The total fat consumption reduced from 37.8% to 28.8%—a 33% reduction. However, a diet obtaining 28.8% of energy from fat cannot be considered a low-fat diet. The stated goal of the study was to reduce that fat to 20% of the calories so that goal was not achieved.
- The amount of saturated fat consumed by the intervention group at 6 years (9.5%) is still higher than the recommended 8%.

- The average dietary fiber intake was 16.9 g after 6 years, which is significantly below the recommendation of 25-30 g/day.
- The goal of the study was to increase fruit and vegetable consumption to 5 servings per day. The achieved average was only 4.9 servings per day.
- The goal was to increase the amount of grain consumption to 6 servings per day. The amount of grains consumed in the intervention group was reduced—not increased.
- The dietary intake was based on self-reporting which has a tendency to be unreliable. Participants are inclined to report findings that support the perceived goals of the researchers.
- The goals for the study are the dietary recommendations for individuals. Ideally, everyone should be reaching these goals. Even if the group average reached the stated goal, there would still be a significant number who failed to reach that goal.

One of the conclusions of this large study was, "that more focused diet and lifestyle interventions may be needed to improve risk factors and reduce CVD risk."

Given that there was so little change in the diet of the intervention group over the six years then it is not surprising that the results did not show a significant reduction in the risk of heart disease and stroke.

There are also ethical issues with this kind of study. For any lifestyle change, participants and their families need to be committed to the concept. Randomly assigning participants to a particular group is not conducive to a positive outcome. Do we really need a random trial that lasts for a number of years, wait for the results to be analyzed and published to validate the hypothesis that diet is an important component of our health?

North Karelia Project

The *Seven Countries Study* highlighted the high death rate, particularly from heart disease, in North Karelia and Finland. North Karelia is an inland region in Eastern Finland that borders Russia.

The *North Karelia Project* is documented in a 300-page document produced by Finland's National Institute for Health and Welfare (THL), in collaboration with the North Karelia Project Foundation.[145]

In 1973, Finland had a highest country death rate for men from cardiac heart disease and North Karelia had the highest rate in Finland.

The difference in mortality rates between East and West Finland had been occurring since the nineteenth century. In the east, prior to World War II, men were often lumberjacks. Diets included game from hunting, picking berries and fishing. Accidents were a health issue as well as tuberculosis and other infectious diseases. After the war, veterans were given small plots of land to farm pigs and cows. Dairy become an important part of the economy and diet.

Henry Blackburn describes a logger's meal in his book *On the Trail of Heart Attacks in the Seven Countries*:[146]

> Loggers' lunches, even today, are things of wonder, unsurpassed in caloric density: Large hunks of meat are suspended in congealed fat, enveloped in a dark bread loaf fully permeated by fat. The whole – at 250 grams of fat and well over 2,000 calories – is packaged in aluminium foil and tied with a ribbon. This hefty fare is preceded by a breakfast of fish soup, containing fifty percent butter fat calories and several grams of salt. The evening meal provides the rest of the 6,000 calories the logger needs to work outdoors all day.

As a direct result of the *Seven Countries Study*, a project, the North Karelia Project, was instigated in 1971. Following its success, the project was expanded to include all of Finland.

Programs centered around anti-smoking, cholesterol lowering nutrition, blood pressure lowering—emphasizing non-pharmacological interventions, weight reduction, and physical and social activities.

Many concerns were expressed over the impact of the dietary changes to the economy. Growing berries as a replacement for dairy was seen as a possibility. Red and black currants, strawberries, and the wild berries growing in the forest areas was a viable opportunity. The Berry Project was conceived in 1985. Local berry consumption has risen with farmers switching from dairy to berry production.

By 2007, the heart disease death rate for men dropped by 80%. Saturated fat intake decreased from 22% of dietary energy intake to 13% and total fat from 38% to 31–32%.

Over the period from 1971 to 2006, life expectancy at birth rose 8.2 years for males and 7.0 years for females.

Although mortality has declined significantly, there is still room for considerable improvement. Smoking rates are still high: in North Karelia—52% of men were smokers in 1972 and 31% in 2007. Despite the significant reduction in fat consumption, consumption of fat is relatively high.

Physicians' Health Study

The *Physicians' Health Study* commenced in 1981. It consisted of a study of 22,071 male doctors between 40 and 84 years of age in the U.S. who reported an absence of heart disease, cancers, liver disease, peptic ulcer, and gout.[147]

The physicians were randomly assigned to one of four groups. One group received aspirin and a beta-carotene supplement, another aspirin with a beta-carotene placebo and a third group an aspirin placebo with a beta-carotene supplement. The fourth group received placebos for both aspirin and the beta-carotene.

The aspirin study ended early since it was determined that aspirin had a significant effect in reducing the risk of myocardial infarction (heart attack).

• • • • •

The *Physicians' Health Study II* tested vitamin C, vitamin E, beta-carotene, and a multivitamin for the primary prevention of cardiovascular disease, total cancer, and prostate cancer. It also evaluated the effect of these agents on colon polyps and colon cancer, cataract, macular degeneration, and early cognitive decline.

Daily multivitamin supplementation modestly reduced the risk of total cancer. The incidence reduced from 18.3 cancer events per 1000 person-years to 17.0 events.

Otherwise, there was no evidence that vitamin E, C or beta-carotene reduced the risk of cancer. None of the interventions reduced the risk of cardiovascular disease.

• • • • •

The role of egg consumption on health was also examined. The result from a 20-year follow-up showed a significant correlation between egg consumption and all-cause mortality.[148]

Egg consumption was divided into 5 categories—less than 1 egg per week, 1 egg per week, 2–4 eggs, 5–6 eggs per week and 7 or more eggs per week.

A key finding is that physicians consuming 7 or more eggs per week had a 31% increase in all-cause mortality compared with those consuming less than 1 egg per week. For diabetic physicians, the association was much higher with the increase in mortality slightly more than doubled.

A British study reported a 2.7 times greater risk of death with an egg consumption greater than 6 eggs per week.[149]

The National Heart Foundation of Australia states that "as part of a healthy balanced diet you can eat up to 6 eggs each week without increasing your risk of heart disease."[150]

Any activity that doubles the mortality rate must be treated with some caution.

Finnish Childhood Diabetes Study

In 1990s, Finland had the highest incidence of diabetes and cow's milk consumption in the world.

In Finland, researchers compared levels of incompletely digested cow's milk protein (Bovine Serum Albumin – BSA) in 142 diabetic children. Levels of IgG anti-BSA antibodies were higher than 3.55 RFUs (relative fluorescence units) for the 142 diabetic children whilst each non-diabetic child in the control group of 79 children had levels of less than 3.55.[151]

There was no overlap of the levels between the two groups of children. All children with diabetes had a higher level of the antibodies (which can only occur from consuming cow's milk) than the group without diabetes.

Significant increases in BSA antibodies in diabetic children have been found in other studies in Finland[152] and France.[153]

• • • • •

A paper[154] published in 1991 compared the incidence rates of insulin-dependent diabetes mellitus (IDDM – Type I diabetes) in children 0–14 years and cow's milk consumption in 12 countries. The countries included were Finland, Sweden, Norway, Great Britain, Denmark, United States, New Zealand, Netherlands, Canada, France, Israel, and Japan.

The coefficient of determination (R^2) was 0.94. The conclusion of the paper was that "the results support the hypothesis that cow's milk may contain a triggering factor for the development of IDDM".

The coefficient of determination is a measure of how well the predicted value approximates the observed data. A value of 1 indicates that the predicted value matches the observed value. In this case, it implies that 94% of the incidence of Type I diabetes may be attributed to dairy consumption.

• • • • •

For Type I diabetes, there is a specific sequence of 17 amino acids that is found in proteins in cow's milk. The immune system recognizes this sequence as a foreign intruder so antibodies are produced to eliminate the unwanted invaders. Unfortunately, the same 17 amino acid sequence is found on the cells of the pancreas that produce insulin. Consequently, the immune system is unable to distinguish the cow's milk protein fragments from the pancreatic cells. It therefore destroys both which leads to the inability of the pancreas to produce insulin and leads to a life time dependency of insulin injections and their consequences.[155]

China-Cornell-Oxford Project

Colin Campbell[156] was a nutritional biochemist at Cornell University. In the 1960s, he was involved in nutritional programs in the Philippines to help families provide for their critically undernourished children. Peanuts were one of their preferred sources of protein. It is a legume—great for improving the soil, easy to grow, and is nutritious and tasty.

At the same time, children younger than 10, were dying at alarming rates from liver cancer. Normally liver cancer is an adult disease—and the children dying from the disease were from the most affluent suburbs in Manilla. These are the families that could afford the best housing and the best food.

Whilst in the Philippines, he read a paper in an obscure medical journal. Rats were fed aflatoxin—one of the deadliest carcinogens known. One group of rats was given a diet of 20% protein —and they all died of liver cancer. The second group was given a diet of 5% protein—and they all lived. 100% deaths compared to zero deaths. They were all fed aflatoxin—but only those rats that had a high protein diet died.

A 20% diet of wheat protein, gluten, or pea protein did not result in liver cancer deaths whereas casein, which comprises of 80% of the protein found in cow's milk, and albumin, which is found in egg white, did result in liver cancer deaths. Plant-based diets are often considered to be lysine deficient. However, adding the amino acid lysine to the wheat protein to match the level found in casein also resulted in cancer deaths.

Significantly, peanuts and corn in the Philippines were often contaminated by aflatoxin—and the wealthy ate Western-style diets, one rich in protein.

A few years later, in the early 1970s, the premier of China, Chen En-lai, was dying of cancer. Late in his life, he instigated a survey of cancers, heart disease, and infectious diseases throughout China. As a result, the *China Atlas* was produced, which shows the mortality rates in more than 2,400 counties. Some regions showed cancer rates over 100 times greater than the counties with the lowest rates.

To study these results, the *China-Cornell-Oxford Project* was formed. The principle researchers were: Colin Campbell, professor of nutritional biochemistry at Cornell; Chen Junshi, Deputy Director of Institute of Nutrition and Food Hygiene at the Chinese Academy of Preventive Medicine in Beijing; Li Junyao of the China Cancer Institute; and the epidemiologist Sir Richard Peto from the University of Oxford. Li Junyao was one of the authors the *China Atlas*. Richard Peto is one of the world's leading epidemiologists.

Surveys were conducted in 1983–1984 and 1989–1990. The study consisted of 6,500 people in 65 counties. In each county, two villages (xiang) were selected with 25 men and 25 women from different families selected from each village. Blood, urine, and food samples were obtained for analysis, questionnaires were completed, and three-day diet information was recorded.

They looked at over 360 different health, lifestyle, and nutrition factors and found over 8,000 significant correlations.

Below are some comparisons of diets in rural China with average American diets.

Nutrient	China[157]				U.S. Percentiles[158]				
	Mean	Min	Median	Max	Mean	5	50	95	1
Energy Intake (kcal/day) M	2609	1707	2608	3578	2567				
Energy Intake (kcal/day) F	2406	1579	2433	3066	1834				
Carbohydrate (g/day) M	476	292	467	740	305	172	303	500	
Carbohydrate (g/day) F	429	256	433	588	228	127	225	361	
Fiber (g/day) M	17.0	4.8	14.0	44.7	20.3	8.5	16.9	31.0	
Fiber (g/day) F	12.7	4.8	11.0	38.8	16.1	6.7	13.5	24.6	
Total Protein (g/day) M	64.6	42.2	64.3	98.7	98.8	60	95	144	2
Total Protein (g/day) F	59.1	40.7	58.1	82.8	68.1	38	63	99	
% Animal / Total Protein M	8.4	0.3	6.8	32.8	70				3
% Animal / Total Protein F	12.2	0	8.6	47.5	66				
% Fat / kcal M	14.6	5.9	14.3	25.4	33.0				
% Fat / kcal F	18.3	7.4	18.4	32.6	32.9				
% Saturated / Total Fat M	11.85	3.27	11.67	28.26	32				
% Saturated / Total Fat F	13.91	5.18	13.23	28.18	32				
Vitamin C (mg/day) M	142.5	10.4	128.3	429.4	92.1	21	77	236	
Vitamin C (mg/day) F	120.2	28.9	111.4	344.9	77.8	27	80	188	
Calcium (mg/day) M	543	241	514	923	1116	423	914	1780	
Calcium (mg/day) F	543	352	519	1056	868	329	613	1167	
Iron (mg/day) M	34.3	17.1	34.3	59.3	18.1	9.5	17.0	30.2	
Iron (mg/day) F	32.5	14.7	32.5	50.6	15.8	7.4	12.5	21.0	

(1) For the China statistics, the minimum and maximum values represent the average of the counties with the lowest and highest values. A percentile of 5% indicates the value, below which 5% of the observations may be found.

(2) The U.S. values calculated from g/kg body weight values using 76 kg weight for males and 61 kg for females.

(3) Of the 65 counties, 42 counties had plant / animal protein ratio of 90% or greater, 27 counties were 95% or greater and 14 counties were 98% or greater.

Even allowing for greater physical activity in China, the Chinese consume more calories but weigh significantly less. Total energy intake in rural China was about 30% higher per kg of body weight than in the U.S. Despite this, obesity was far less prevalent in China than in the U.S.

Iron consumption was much greater in the Chinese population, despite consuming less animal products. Fiber intake is significantly higher whilst fat, protein, and animal-based foods are less.

Breast cancer is much less common in rural China. It was significantly associated with dietary fat and higher levels of reproductive hormones such as estrogen and testosterone as a result of high meat and dairy rich diets found in Western countries.

The *China-Cornell-Oxford Project*[159] shows that a higher level of dietary fat and animal-based foods is associated with higher blood cholesterol. These factors are associated with a higher life-time exposure to female hormones, which are associated with more breast cancer and earlier age of menarche. The range for the villages in the study was fifteen to nineteen years, with an average of seventeen years. The U.S. average was about eleven years.

These findings also support the idea that young girls on Western-style diets reach menarche more quickly due to increased growth rates. They sustain higher levels of steroid hormones during their reproductive years, extend their time for menopause, and incur a higher risk of breast cancer.

Colon and rectum cancers in China are much less common than in the United States. These cancers are associated with lower intakes of a wide variety of dietary fiber components only found in plant based foods.

Stomach cancer is much more common in China than in the U.S. because of the effects of *Helicobacter pylori* infection upon the stomach wall. This bacteria is also associated with stomach ulcers.

Liver cancer is about 30 times more common in China than the U.S. due to hepatitis infections.

The consumption of animal products and subsequent increase of blood cholesterol levels result in a higher level of IGF-1 related cancer risk.

One of the chief findings was its significant correlation with breast cancer mortality with dietary fat over a range of 6-24% of calories consumed, although this range is much less than that of Western countries. Even at this relatively low range, the greater the consumption of fat, the higher the incidence of breast cancer.

Other significant findings are the positive association of animal protein with blood cholesterol (both total and LDL) and the inverse association with blood cholesterol and with plant protein.

7

History of Dieting

Low-Carbohydrate Diets

William Banting was a very overweight English carpenter and undertaker. He consulted "other high orthodox authorities (never any inferior adviser), but all in vain."

Eventually, in August of 1862, Banting consulted a noted Fellow of the Royal College of Surgeons—an ear, nose, and throat specialist, Dr William Harvey. As a result of his experience, he wrote a successful pamphlet, *Letter on Corpulence*,[160] in which he describes his experience.

> I am now nearly 66 years of age, about 5 feet 5 inches [165 cm] in stature, and, in August last (1862), weighed 202 lbs. [92 kg].

Over a period of 12 months, he lost 46 pounds (21 kg) resulting in a weight of 167 pounds (76 kg). It was a big improvement but not exactly slim. His recipe for achieving this is:

For breakfast, I take four or five ounces of beef, mutton, kidneys, broiled fish, bacon, or cold meat of any kind except pork; a large cup of tea (without milk or sugar), a little biscuit, or one ounce of dry toast.

For dinner. Five or six ounces of any fish except salmon, any meat except pork, any vegetable except potato, one ounce of dry toast, fruit out of a pudding, any kind of poultry or game, and two or three glasses of good claret, sherry, or Madeira - Champagne, Port and Beer forbidden.

For tea. Two or three ounces of fruit, a rusk or two, and a cup of tea without milk or sugar.

For supper. Three or four ounces of meat or fish, similar to dinner, with a glass or two of claret.

For nightcap, if required, A tumbler of grog - (gin, whisky, or brandy, without sugar) or a glass or two of claret or sherry.

This plan leads to an excellent night's rest, with from six to eight hours' sound sleep. The dry toast or rusk may have a table spoonful of spirit to soften it, which will prove acceptable.

Perhaps I did not wholly escape starchy or saccharine [sugar] matter, but scrupulously avoided those beans, such as milk, sugar, beer, butter, &c., which were known to contain them.

Shortly after the First World War, the large American chemical firm E.I. DuPont, became concerned about the growing obesity problem among their staff. They hired Dr Alfred Pennington to find out why traditional low-calorie diets were not working.

Basing his program on the work of Pittsburgh doctor, Frank Evans[161], Dr Pennington placed DuPont executives on a high-fat, high-protein, low-carbohydrate, unrestricted-calorie diet.[162] His dieters reported they felt well, enjoyed their meals, and were never hungry between meals. The 20 obese individuals he treated lost an average of 10 kg each, in an average time of three-and-a-half months.

This is based on the theory that people become fat because they cannot fully break down carbohydrates and so they become converted to fat.[163]

• • • • •

Robert Atkins[164] was born in 1930 in Dayton, Ohio. He received an undergraduate degree from the University of Michigan in 1951 and earned a medical degree from Cornell University. His cardiology residency was obtained at St. Luke's Hospital, New York. At the age of 33, he had his picture taken for an ID. He told *Observer Food Monthly*, "I looked at a picture of myself and realized I had a triple chin. [...] I was eating junk food. Nobody had ever told me junk food was bad for me. Four years of medical school, and four years of internship and residency, and I never thought anything was wrong with eating sweet rolls and doughnuts, and potatoes, and bread, and sweets."

An article examining Pennington's work, titled *A New Concept in the Treatment of Obesity*,[165] was published in 1963, and advocated for the complete elimination of sugar from the diet and a marked increase in both fat and protein. Atkins had recently read the article in the journal. He says, 'It was so simple! I hadn't tried a diet before that. It was the only diet that looked like I'd enjoy being on it. I ate a lot of meat, and a lot of shrimp, and a lot of duck, and a lot of fish. And omelettes in the morning, and salad and vegetables.'

Atkins lost 12 kg in six weeks on a low-carbohydrate diet. 100% of his 65 patients who trialed the diet reached their target weights.

In 1970, he wrote an article for *Vogue* on his low-carbohydrate. In 1972, he published his book, *Dr Atkins' Diet Revolution*, which sold 15 million copies. His program was condemned by the American Medical Association. It is a remarkable outcome, given that he originally obtained the idea from the association's journal.

Atkins died at the age of 72 in New York in 2003, after falling on ice. His report was mistakenly released to the public. The report suggested that Atkins had "a history of heart attack, congestive heart failure and hypertension." It also states that his death was caused by a "blunt impact injury of head" and records his weight and height at 258 pounds [117 kg] and 6 feet [182 cm] tall, which is classed as "obese". At the request of his family, an autopsy was not performed. His supporters state Atkins suffered from cardiomyopathy, which was likely caused by a virus.[166]

• • • • •

Dr Barry Sears is the author and co-author of the approximately 20 *Zone Diet* books: *Enter the Zone* (1995); *Mastering the Zone* (1996); *The Zone Diet* (1999); *The 7-day Zone Diet* (2003); and *A Week in the Zone* (2004). He is a former research scientist at the Boston University School of Medicine and the Massachusetts Institute of Technology.

According to Sears,[167] "being overweight or obese is not your fault. [...] It is due to the adverse interaction of your genes with radical changes that have taken place in the American diet over the past twenty-five years." Also, "for every *one* gram of fat you eat, you want *two* grams of protein, and *three* grams of carbohydrates." This equates to obtaining approximately 40% of energy from carbohydrates, 30% protein, and 30% fat.

Sears claims, "the underlying cause of chronic disease comes from the increased production of a natural fatty acid called arachidonic acid which is incredibly toxic at high enough concentrations." He states, "the most likely suspect gene-altering drama is increased consumption of omega-6 fatty acids, such as linoleic acid, which lower the percentage of omega-3 fats in the diet." and "we have been become genetically altered by increasing linoleic acid to gain weight rapidly and make it difficult to lose."[168] Arachidonic acid is abundant in the brain, muscles, and liver.

Supplements in the form of fish oils, to supply omega-3 fatty acids, and proprietary-brand polyphenols are "required to manage diet-induced inflammation for a lifetime."

The advice includes, "add a lot colorful vegetables and a little fruit. Fruits and vegetables to avoid are those that are high in sugar (e.g., bananas, carrots, grapes, raisins) or starchy (e.g., potatoes, corn)." It is suggested that grains, being starch foods, should be kept to a minimum.[169]

• • • • •

Cardiologist Arthur Agatston and dietitian Marie Almon created the *South Beach Diet* in the 1980s as an alternative to low-fat approaches advocated by the American Heart Association.

This is a 3 phase dietary plan which is summarized below.[170]

Phase 1: First 2 weeks eat healthy, lean protein (fish, shellfish, chicken, turkey, and lean meats), loads of vegetables and salads, nuts, reduced-fat cheeses, low-fat dairy and good unsaturated olive and canola oil.

Avoid starches (bread, rice, pasta) and sugars (fruit and fruit juices).

Phase 2: Followed until you hit your target weight. Add back the foods you love, like the "good" carbohydrates – fruit, whole-grain bread, whole-grain rice, whole-wheat pasta, and sweet potatoes (no white potatoes). Avoid high-glycemic foods.

If phase 2 fails then return to phase 1.

Phase 3: Avoid bad fats and bad carbohydrates. Good fats are unsaturated fats. Limit the amount of omega-6 fatty acids. Good carbohydrates are low-glycemic carbohydrates.

• • • • •

Pierre Dukan[171] is a French medical doctor, initially specializing in neurology. Since 1973, he has been involved with nutrition. The *Dukan Diet* book was published in 2000 with a four-phase dietary plan.

According to the official Dukan website, "Dr Pierre Dukan has identified 100 ingredients to be eaten as much as you want in your Dukan Diet meal plan. They are low in lipids (fat) and carbohydrates (sugar), and high in protein and other nutritional elements essential to the body's well-being."

Beefsteak, chicken and a number of cold water fish are included in the "Eat As Much As You Want Foods" list.

Oat bran is a cornerstone of the Dukan Diet.

• • • • •

Gastroenterologist Walter Voegtlin published a book, *The Stone Age Diet* that proposed a diet "based on in-depth Studies of Human Ecology and the Diet of Man". According to this book:

> Did anybody ever tell you that your ancestors were exclusively carnivores for at least two and possibly twenty million years? Were you aware

that ancestral man first departed slightly from a strictly carnivorous diet a mere ten thousand years ago?[172]

The idea was developed by Dr Stanley Boyd Eaton and Dr Melvin Konner. Eaton, a radiologist, graduated from Harvard Medical School in 1964. Konner is a medical doctor and anthropologist. He is currently (2016) a professor of anthropology at Emory University in Atlanta.

Their initial paper *Paleolithic Nutrition - A Consideration of Its Nature and Current Implications* was published in the *New England Journal* in 1985.[173] This was followed by the book, *The Paleolithic Prescription*[174] in 1988 which was written by Eaton, Konner and Marjorie Shostak.

The premise is that early humans, from 1.8–1.6 million years ago, began to consume a much larger quantity of meat than their hominid ancestors, who mainly consumed fruit.

Dr Loren Cordain is a professor at the Department of Health and Exercise Science at Colorado State University. He published the book, *The Paleo Diet* (2001) that promoted the concept and helped popularize the diet. He obtained his Ph.D. in exercise physiology from University of Utah in 1981.[175]

Permissible foods are meat and poultry (grass-fed and free-ranging), fish and other sea foods, eggs, vegetables, fruit, nuts, seeds, and "healthy" oils. Foods to avoid include all dairy, grains, processed foods, potatoes, refined sugar, salt, refined vegetable oils, and legumes.[176] Paleolithic diets are high in protein (19-35% of energy requirements) and fats (28-47%) and low in carbohydrates (22-40%).[177]

• • • • •

Terry Wahls is a medical doctor and clinical professor of medicine at University of Iowa Carver College of Medicine in Iowa City, Iowa, U.S. She was diagnosed with multiple sclerosis in 2000. Twelve months after being confined to a wheel chair in 2007, she was able to ride a bike 18 miles (29 km). Part of her rehabilitation included a modified hunter-gather diet.

A trial to study the results of interventions for patients with multiple sclerosis reported significant improvement in fatigue. The interventions included a modified paleolithic diet with supplements, stretching, strengthening exercises with electrical stimulation of trunk and lower limb muscles, meditation, and massage.[178]

Ten subjects started the study. Eight completed the study and six subjects fully adhered the interventions for twelve months. It is a diet high in fruit and vegetables and very high in protein (110 g of animal protein and 110 g of plant protein). Dairy and eggs are excluded.

Given the number of interventions, it is not possible to determine the impact of diet in the significant improvement of the 60% of the patients that fully participated in the trial.

• • • • •

Dr Katharine Milton is a professor of physical anthropology at the University of California in Berkeley. She received her Ph.D. in anthropology from New York University in 1977.

Her field of expertise is the dietary ecology of primates, including human ancestors and modern humans.

According to Professor Milton:

> In fact, we do not know much about the range of foods Paleolithic hunter-gatherers consumed in almost any environment.[179]

Comparative and experimental data shows that modern humans, common chimpanzees, gorillas, and orangutans show close similarity to most features of gut anatomy as well as patterns of digestive kinetics.[180]

Most monkeys and apes include considerable amount of fruit in their diet. These fruit are more nutritious than cultivated fruits. Wild fruits are higher in protein, minerals, vitamins, and fiber and have less fat. They are higher in omega-3 fatty acids. Wild fruits are also higher in glucose and fructose but lower in sucrose. Sucrose is a disaccharide which contains a molecule of glucose and fructose which needs to be broken down into the component parts before it can be utilized by humans.[181]

All primates obtain the majority of their food from plant sources. Primates include lemurs, monkeys, apes, and humans. Examples include the following species.[182]

Primate	Scientific name	Plant sourced food
African blue monkey	Cercopithecus mitis	73%
Red-tailed monkey	Cercopithecus ascanius	75%
Baboon	Papio spp	> 90%
Rhesus macaques	Macacca mulatta	> 99%
Howler monkeys	Alouatla spp	99%
Spider monkeys	Atteles spp	97%
Orangutan	Pongo pygmaeus	97%
Gorilla	Gorilla gorilla	97%
Chimpanzee	Pan troglodyles	88.5 - ≥ 95%

One difference is that chimpanzees, bonobos, and orangutans produce less of the enzyme amylase than human populations. Amylase is the most abundant protein in human saliva and is required to breakdown starches into the component simple sugar—glucose.

Professor Milton's conclusion is:

> It is prudent for modern-day humans to remember their long evolutionary heritage as anthropoid primates and heed current recommendations to increase the number and variety of fresh fruit and vegetables in their diets rather than increase their intake of domesticated animal fat and protein[183]

• • • • •

The naturopath James D'Adamo developed the Blood Type Diet based on the principle your diet should be determined by your blood type. According to this system:

- From 40,000 to 30,000 years ago "humans thrived on meat" and adding the assumption that blood type-O is the oldest blood type then people with blood type-O should be eating a high-protein, meat-based diet.
- Type-A blood group appeared in Asia or the Middle East between 25,000 and 15,000 BC in response to new environmental conditions. Due to the cultivation of grains and livestock, type-A blood group was created. Type-A is a vegetarian-based diet.
- Type-B developed between 10,000 and 15,000 BC in the area now a part of Pakistan and India. Type-B is a "balanced omnivore" eating meat (no chicken), dairy, grains, beans, legumes, vegetables, and fruit.

According to researchers led by Laure Segurel of the University of Chicago, the A and B blood groups evolved at least 20 million years ago and are shared by humans, bonobos, chimpanzees, gorillas, orangutans, gibbons, and several species of monkeys. Blood type-O (which is the absence of type-A or type-B antigens) appeared at a later stage.[184]

Subsequently, D'Adamo's son, Peter, has further developed the diet. He has added a refinement, the Genotype Diet, based on six genotypes that relates diet to blood groups, personality, and body type. The six categories of the Genotype Diet are: Hunter; Gatherer; Teacher; Explorer; Warrior; and Nomad. The concept that personality and blood groups are related originated in Japan in the 1920s.[185]

A study involving 1,455 participants published in 2014, showed that those adhering to a type-A diet had an improvement in their cardiac and metabolic risk profiles, but this was independent of their blood group. The type-A diet emphasizes a high consumption of fruits and vegetables, and low consumption of meat products.[186]

Standard Western Diet

In the United States, the average protein intake (as a percentage of calories) is 16% with a range of 10% to 22%.[187]

The average fat intake is 34% (as a percentage of calories) with 11% of the calories coming from saturated fats.

Simple sugars comprise of 44% of the total carbohydrates with dietary fiber making up 6%.

Meat consumption per person is at a record high with an increase 40% since the 1950s.

• • • • •

On January 2016, the DASH Diet was "ranked best diet for 6th year in a row by US News & World Report."[188]

Several studies, originating from Harvard School of Public Health, relating diet and blood pressure were published during 1970s and 1980s. These studies showed:

The declared consumption of food of animal origin was highly significantly associated with systolic and diastolic BP after the age and weight effects were removed.[189]

In recent investigation of blood-pressure levels in a group of vegetarians, who were following a macrobiotic diet, levels of diastolic and systolic pressure were found to be relatively low and significantly and positively associated with the amount of animal products ingested.[190]

The study suggests an adverse effect of consumption of beef on plasma lipid and BP levels.[191]

Vegetarians have lower BP than do non-vegetarians in the United States and Australia.[192]

In 1997, the results of the *Dietary Approaches to Stop Hypertension* (DASH) trial was published. This trial tested three types of diet with 459 people with elevated blood pressure to study the effects of diet on blood pressure. The participants with high blood pressure were excluded. Participants were randomly assigned to one of the three diets for an eight-week period. Normal blood pressure levels were defined as: systolic measurement less than 120 mmHg; and diastolic measurement less than 80 mmHg.[193]

The control diet was "typical of the diets of a substantial number of Americans". The fruits-and-vegetables diet provided "more fruits and vegetables and fewer snacks and sweets than the control diet but was otherwise similar to it".

The combination diet was "rich in fruits, vegetables, and low-fat dairy foods and had reduced amounts of saturated fat, total fat, and cholesterol." This experimental diet was labelled "ideal".

Compared with the control diet, the combination diet reduced systolic blood pressure by an average of 5.5 mmHg and the fruits-and-vegetables diet reduced systolic blood pressure by 2.8 mmHg.

Below is a comparison of the control diet, with the "fruits and vegetables" diet and the "ideal combination" diet. The amount of food is measured in grams per day.[194]

Food groups	Control g/day	Fruit & veg g/day	Combo diet g/day
Red meat (beef, pork, lamb and veal)	95	108	24
Meat (red meat, fish, poultry)	192	172	139
Vegetables	147	272	345
Dairy products	89	59	485
Fats and oils	54	43	26
Sweets and sugar containing snacks	152	28	22

The fruits-and-vegetables diet had a higher intake of red meat than the other two diets and a greater intake of total meat than the combination diet. The combination diet had more vegetables than the fruits-and-vegetables diet. The DASH diet is a high-protein, high-fat diet compared to the vegetarian diets that were evaluated during the 1970s and 1980s.

The American Heart Association has similar guidelines. Their recommendations include eating oily fish at least twice a week. As discussed earlier, there is ample evidence to suggest that fish oil or omega-3 oil supplements are not protective of heart disease.[195]

Below is a table that shows the daily nutrient goals used in the DASH studies and a comparison with the average US Diet.[196 197]

Nutrient	US Diet	DASH Diet
Total fat	34% of calories	27% of calories
Saturated fat	11% of calories	6% of calories
Protein	16% of calories	15% of calories
Carbohydrate	50% of calories	58% of calories

A study published in 2014, documented the changes of participants who consumed a whole-food, plant-based diet with no added oils. After seven days, the median reduction for participants with elevated systolic blood pressure (140 mmHg or greater) was 18 mmHg and 4 mmHg for those with "normal" blood pressure.[198] (The median is the 50th percentile—half the participants had a greater reduction and half had a smaller reduction.)

When people, who are eating a standard Western diet, embark on a low-fat diet, a frequent outcome is: an increase in protein consumption; an increase in cholesterol consumption (as a result of eating more fish and "low-fat" dairy); and the proportion of animal-based foods consumed increases to 80-85%. This is due to an increase in low-fat dairy products, fish and egg consumption.

Mediterranean Diets

There are approximately 25 countries that border the Mediterranean Sea. These countries vary greatly in culture, customs, and diet. The Mediterranean diet refers to the traditional diets of Spain, Greece and southern Italy. The *Seven Countries Study* examined the diets of southern Italy and Greece during the late 1950s and early 1960s. This period was sufficiently removed from the constraints of World War II but the influence of western fast food outlets had not yet made an impact.

A healthy Mediterranean diet is mainly vegetarian and is much lower in meat and dairy products than American and northern European diets. Fruit is commonly eaten for dessert.

According to Ancel Keys, who originated the term, the Mediterranean diet consists of "pasta in many forms, leaves sprinkled with olive oil, all kinds of vegetables in season, and often cheese, all finished off with fruit, and frequently washed down with wine."[199]

Later researchers concluded that traditional Mediterranean diet has eight components:[200] [201]

- high monounsaturated to saturated fat ratio—the main fat consumed is olive oil
- moderate alcohol consumption, consumed with meals
- high consumption of legumes
- high consumption of cereals (including bread)

- high consumption of fruits
- high consumption of vegetables
- low consumption of meat and meat products
- minimal consumption of milk and dairy products

In recent decades, the amount of meat and dairy consumed has risen in Italy, Greece and Spain.

The National Geographic has being involved in longevity studies since the 1970s. Two Mediterranean regions have been studied extensively as part of their Blue Zones project.

The mountainous region of Barbagia in central Sardinia has the highest concentrations of male centenarians on the planet. The ratio of female to male centenarians is 1:1 where in most places it is 4:1.[202] Diet in the Barbagia region is essentially a plant-based diet that includes potatoes, bread made from whole wheat or barley flour, fava beans, and garden vegetables. Sheep or goat cheese is also consumed. Minestrone (a vegetable soup) is commonly eaten. Meat is consumed possibly once a week. Wine also is regularly consumed with meals. Since Barbagia is an inland, mountainous region, only limited amounts of fish is consumed.

Ikaria, a Greek island in the eastern Aegean Sea, is another Mediterranean location whose inhabitants are frequently studied for their health and longevity. It is also a mountainous region. Ikaria inhabitants have a more varied diet than those in Barbagia, Sardinia. Components of their diet include bread from whole-grain cereal, potatoes, beans (garbanzo, black-eyed peas, and lentils), and an abundance of garden vegetables and greens with liberal amounts of olive oil. Goat milk is also consumed. Alcohol is served daily with meals with fish eaten only in small amounts. Meat is served possibly once a week. Fruit consumption is relatively low.

Both in Barbagia and Sardinia, potatoes and bread are a valuable part of the diet. These two items have received poor publicity in recent dietary commentaries.

Whole-Food, Plant-Based Diets

Possibly one of the first documents extolling the virtues of whole foods instead of processed foods was published in 1847 by Dr Daniel Carr of Birmingham, England. His pamphlet, *The necessity of brown bread for digestion, nourishment, and sound health, and the injurious effects of white bread*, advocates the use of coarse-ground wholemeal flour for making bread instead of superfine white flour:

> It is clear then that the coarser parts of the wheat when ground should never be separated from the fine, at least only the very coarsest parts; but both should be allowed to remain together, then made into bread in the ordinary manner. [...] If habitually employed, together with other precautions, would render medicine comparatively useless for the cure of almost every symptom connected with indigestion. I scarcely ever knew a single case, in which attention was paid to this particular, that did not receive radical benefit and regain a proper tone of the stomach

and alimentary canal.— It never fails with my patients who adopt it.[203]

Carr also refers to Professor Francois Magendie (1783–1855), who fed dogs white bread and water, with all the animals dying within 50 days. All animals fed bread containing bran "continued to thrive on it very well".

• • • • •

Nathan Pritikin[204] was born in Chicago in 1915. He spent his early life as an engineer and inventor. He was diagnosed with coronary artery disease in his early forties. In response to his condition, he developed his low-fat, low-cholesterol, high-carbohydrate diet. He was able to lower his own cholesterol from 280 mg/dL (5.4 mmol/L) to below 150 mg/dL (3.9 mmol/L). His diet was essentially a whole-food, plant-based diet with the addition of small amounts of skim milk products, lean beef, chicken, and fish (small amounts).

Pritikin stated that he included meat "because he figured out what he thought would be the minimal amount of animal product required to meet the needs for B12 without having to supplement." He also included dairy, "to make sure he had some customers and did not want to scare everyone away".

• • • • •

Dr John McDougall published a paper that described the effects of consuming a whole-food, plant-based diet. The diet consisted of no animal-derived products or isolated vegetable oils. Meals included wheat flour products, corn, rice, oats, barley, quinoa, potatoes, sweet potatoes, beans, peas, lentils, fresh fruits and non-starchy green, orange, and yellow vegetables. The macro nutrient profile was approximately 7% fat, 12% protein, and 81% carbohydrate by energy consumption.

After seven days, there was a substantial reduction to relevant bio-markers. The reduction occurred even though 86% of patients on blood pressure medications and 90% of patients on diabetes medications reduced their dosage or discontinued the medication.

Decrease in	Median	Interquartile Range (IQR)
Weight	1.4 kg	1.8 kg
Cholesterol	22 mg/dL (0.6 mmol/L)	29 mg/dL (0.75 mmol/L)
Systolic BP	8 mmHg	18 mmHg
Diastolic BP	4 mmHg	10 mmHg
Blood glucose	3 mg/dL (0.2 mmol/L)	11 mg/dL (0.6 mmol/L)

Note: The median is the midpoint value. 50% of the participants experienced a greater change and 50% experienced a smaller change. The IQR is the range of the middle 50% of the measurements.

• • • • •

Dr James Anderson is Emeritus Professor at the University of Kentucky who has been researching diabetes for more than 30 years. He advocates a high-carbohydrate, high-fiber diet for treating diabetes.

Ideally, diets providing 70% of calories as carbohydrate and up to 70 gm fiber daily offer the greatest health benefits for individuals with diabetes. However, these diets allow only one to two ounces of meat daily and are impractical for home use for many individuals.[205]

It should be noted that living with diabetes is not always practical either.

• • • • •

William Roberts is a leading cardiovascular pathologist. He is the current editor (at 2016) of the *American Journal of Cardiology*—a position he has held since 1982. He has published over 1,500 articles. Roberts served as the first head of the pathology service at the National Heart, Lung, and Blood Institute at the National Institutes of Health from 1964 to 1993. He has been located at Baylor Heart and Vascular Institute and Baylor University Medical Center in Dallas, Texas since 1993.

Dr Roberts wrote an editorial titled, *We think we are one, we act as if we are one, but we are not one*. He was referring to us thinking that we are "carnivores". His conclusion is:

> Although we think we are one and act as if we were one, human beings are not natural carnivores. When we kill animals to eat them, they end up killing us because their flesh […] was never intended for human beings […].[206]

Carnivores have claws to hunt prey, smaller stomach and intestines, synthesize vitamin C, lap water, have sharper teeth, and have stronger jaws. Try catching a buffalo or a mammoth with your bare hands and making a meal out of the carcass without tools.

Dr Roberts has also suggested cholesterol goals should be less than 150 mg/dL for total cholesterol and less than 60 mg/dL for LDL cholesterol. He also contends there is only one risk factor for heart disease—that is, "It's the cholesterol, stupid", [207] and that the HDL-cholesterol is largely irrelevant.

8

Conclusion

This book arose from a formal complaint written by the author in response to a television program. Two episodes of the *Heart of the Matter* series were presented by *Catalyst*, a program produced in Australia by the Australian Broadcasting Corporation (ABC). The first episode argued that saturated fats and cholesterol was not involved in coronary vascular disease. The second episode argued that statin drugs were not an appropriate treatment for people with elevated blood cholesterol levels.

My complaint concerned the accuracy of the material presented by the first episode. However, the conclusion of the review process stated that "no material inaccuracy has been demonstrated by any complainant."[208] The intention of this book is to demonstrate that substantial errors did arise in many instances throughout the *Catalyst* program.

The report also stated that "the program did not explicitly endorse the unorthodox view" that saturated fat and heart disease are not linked. The following statement made at the beginning of the program clearly is an endorsement of the unorthodox view.

> I will follow the road which lead us to believe that saturated fat and cholesterol cause heart disease and reveal why it is being touted as the biggest myth in medical history.

Most of the 146 complaints received by the ABC concerned the second episode relating to treatment of heart disease by the prescription of statin drugs.

The complaint against the second episode, *Cholesterol Drug War*, was upheld. The reason given was that "the principal relevant perspective that statins have wider benefits for this group was not properly presented."

The mechanism of cholesterol manufacture in the body is well understood. Statins work by inhibiting mevalonate formation. Since mevalonate is produced during the synthesis of cholesterol then cholesterol production is reduced. This results in an increase in the number of LDL receptors on liver cell membranes and increases the ability of the liver cells to extract cholesterol from the blood.

If statins do have a benefits for a "certain group of people", it is only because high levels of cholesterol is implicated in heart disease. It is difficult to comprehend how the review considered statins to be important for the treatment of heart disease whilst believing that there is a "compelling case to cast doubt over the intense focus that has been given to the role of cholesterol in heart disease".

· · · · ·

It is disturbing to read and hear gossip regarding people such as Ancel Keys, Colin Campbell and George McGovern that completely misrepresent their life's work.

It does not require much investigation to discover that Ancel Keys did not "cherry-pick" his data. The statement that "there was data available from 22 countries and Keys only chose those six (or seven) that confirmed his hypothesis" is found in numerous publications. Unfortunately, not one of these commentators have stated the source of the data for these 22 countries. The mostly likely source was a paper published in 1957 by Jacob Yerushalmy and Herman Hilleboe.[209] This paper showed data from 22 countries that was sourced from the *Food and Agriculture Organization* of the United Nations for the years 1951-1953. Keys's paper was first presented at a conference in Amsterdam in late 1952.[210] It was later presented on 7 January 1953 at Mt Sinai Hospital in New York. This is the paper that was published and commonly referenced.[211] Clearly, the data from these 22 counties was not available at the time Keys's paper was written.

Another comment that is frequently made by the same commentators is that Keys could have chosen another six (or seven) countries that would give different results. Which countries? As stated previously, Yerushalmy and Hilleboe did find significant correlations with different components of the diet and heart disease—even when all 22 countries were considered.

•••••

The food we eat is a complex combination of many components—many different types of fat, carbohydrates, amino acids, and dietary fiber along with a multitude of micro-nutrients including vitamins, minerals, carotenoids, and polyphenols. Focusing on one component such as saturated fats or cholesterol may help understand some elements of health. However, the complex interaction between even two or three components make it impossible to fully comprehend the effects of nutrition in real life. Most medical and nutritional studies are only concerned with the effects of one dietary component or intervention.

Our health is related to many interrelated factors and is not limited to what we eat—although, an imbalance of a single dietary element may have profound effects, either beneficial or otherwise. Other elements of our lives have a profound impact on our well-being:

- close family relationships—including our pets
- the ability to breathe properly affects every aspect of health
- relationship with our community and society
- quality of our water
- infectious diseases
- having a purpose and goals that reflect our values
- our relationship with the environment
- financial security
- exercise and physical activity

All of these factors greatly influence our ability to live a full and healthy life.

9

Suggested Reading

Daniel Steinberg is a researcher the field of lipid metabolism and atherosclerosis. He discovered the role of low-density lipoprotein oxidation in the development of atherosclerosis. He wrote a comprehensive account of the history of cardiovascular research *The Cholesterol Wars - The Skeptics vs. the Preponderance of Evidence.*[212]

Stewart Truswell was a full time researcher on coronary heart disease at the MRC Atheroma Research Unit in Glasgow, directed by Dr Brian Bronte-Stewart. The unit closed when Dr Bronte-Stewart died aged 39. Professor Truswell was an academic general physician in Cape Town, then professor of human nutrition at London University then at Sydney University. John Yudkin was his predecessor at London University. His book is *Cholesterol and Beyond: The Research on Diet and Coronary Heart Disease 1900-2000.*[213]

He also wrote the book *ABC of Nutrition*, published by the British Medical Journal.[214]

Professor Truswell and Professor Jim Mann of University of Otago edited the book, *Essentials of Human Nutrition*.[215]

Joseph Dixon is a lipid biochemist, cell biologist and an Associate Professor of Nutrition in the Department of Nutritional Sciences at Rutgers University, New Brunswick. He wrote a short biography of Ancel and Margaret Keys—*Genius and Partnership: Ancel and Margaret Keys and the Discovery of the Mediterranean Diet*.[216]

Endnotes

1   Lustig, R. (2013) *Fat Chance: Beating the Odds Against Sugar, Processed Food, Obesity, and Disease*. New York: Penguin Group.

2   Boulding, C. (2012) *The Men Who Made Us Fat*.

3   Truswell, A. S. (2010) *Cholesterol and Beyond: The Research on Diet and Coronary Heart Disease 1900-2000*. Springer Netherlands.

4   Keys, A. et al. (1980) *Seven Countries: A Multivariate Analysis of Death and Coronary Heart Disease*. Cambridge, Massachusetts and London, England: Harvard University Press, 335.

5   Keys, A. (1971) Sucrose in the Diet and Coronary Heart Disease. *Atherosclerosis*. 14 (1), 193–202.

6   Demasi, M. & Arnott, I. (2013) *Heart of the Matter - Part 1*.

7   Eades, M. (n.d.) *Experts in the science of low-carb nutrition - The official website of Drs. Michael & Mary Dan Eades* [online]. Available from: https://proteinpower.com/experts-in-the-science-of-low-carb-nutrition/ (Accessed 31 August 2015).

8   Bowden, J. (n.d.) *Jonny Bowden | The Nutrition Mythbuster – Meet Jonny Bowden, PhD, CNS* [online]. Available from: http://jonnybowden.com/meet-jonny-bowden/ (Accessed 31 August 2015).

9   Sinatra, S. (n.d.) *About Dr. Sinatra* [online]. Available from: http://www.drsinatra.com/about-dr-sinatra/ (Accessed 31 August 2015).

10 Taubes, G. (n.d.) *Gary Tabues - Biography* [online]. Available from: http://garytaubes.com/biography/ (Accessed 31 August 2015).

11 Keys, A. (1953) Atherosclerosis: a problem in newer public health. *Journal of Mt Sinai Hospital.* July-Aug; 20 (2), 118–139.

12 Yerushalmy, J. & Hilleboe, H. E. (1957) *Fat in the Diet and Mortality from Heart Disease.*

13 Keys, A. (1995) Mediterranean diet and public health : personal reflections. *American Journal of Clinical Nutrition.* 1321S-1323S.

14 Yudkin, J. (1972) *Pure, White and Deadly: the problem of sugar.* London: Davis-Poynter Limited.

15 Truswell, A. S. (2010) *Cholesterol and Beyond: The Research on Diet and Coronary Heart Disease 1900-2000.* Springer Netherlands.

16 Keys, A. (1971) Sucrose in the Diet and Coronary Heart Disease. *Atherosclerosis.* 14 (1), 200.

17 de Lorgeril, M. et al. (1999) Mediterranean diet, traditional risk factors, and the rate of cardiovascular complications after myocardial infarction: final report of the Lyon Diet Heart Study. *Circulation.* 99 (6), 779–785.

18 Mills, B. K. (1980) The Nutritionist Who Prepared the Pro-Cholesterol Report Defends It Against Critics. People Magazine [online]. Available from: http://www.people.com/people/archive/article/0,,20076734,00.html.

19 Campbell, T. C. & Campbell, T. M. (2006) *The China Study.* Dallas USA: Benbella Books, 258.

20 Armstrong, J. (2014) *If Only: George McGovern and the America That Might Have Been.* North Berwick ME USA: PSA Communications.

21 Campbell, T. C. & Campbell, T. M. (2006) *The China Study.* Dallas USA: Benbella Books, 252.

22 Keys, A. & Keys, M. (1959) *Eat Well and Stay Well.* Doubleday, Garden City, NY.

23 Keys, A. & Keys, M. (1967) *The Benevolent Bean.* New York: Doubleday, Garden City, NY.

24 Keys, A. & Keys, M. (1975) *How to eat well and stay well the Mediterranean way.* Doubleday, Garden City, NY.

25 Walsh, B. (2014) Don't Blame Fat. TIME Magazine 183 (24) p.16–23.

26 Blackburn, H. W. (1995) *On the Trail of Heart Attacks in Seven Countries*. Minnesota: University of Minnesota. [online]. Available from: http://sph.umn.edu/site/docs/epi/SPH%20 Seven%20Countries%20Study.pdf (Accessed 3 June 2016). (Accessed 3 June 2016).

27 Kromhout, D. et al. (1989) Food consumption patterns in the 1960s in seven countries. *American Journal of Clinical Nutrition*. 49 (5), 889–894.

28 Keys, A. et al. (1980) *Seven Countries: A Multivariate Analysis of Death and Coronary Heart Disease*. Cambridge, Massachusetts and London, England: Harvard University Press, 9, 65, 252.

29 Teicholz, N. (2014) *The Big Fat Surprise: why butter, meat, and cheese belong in a healthy diet*. Revised Edition. Scribe.

30 Steinberg, D. (2007) *The Cholesterol Wars: The Skeptics vs. the Preponderance of Evidence*. San Diego, CA: Academic Press.

31 Truswell, A. S. (2010) *Cholesterol and Beyond: The Research on Diet and Coronary Heart Disease 1900-2000*. Springer Netherlands.

32 Dobbin, E. V. et al. (1951) *The Low-Fat, Low-Cholesterol Diet*. Doubleday, Garden City, NY.

33 Rinzler, S. H. (1968) Primary prevention of coronary heart disease by diet. *Bulletin of the New York Academy of Medicine*. 44 (8), 938.

34 Christakis, G. et al. (1966) The anti-coronary club. A dietary approach to the prevention of coronary heart disease–a seven-year report. *American Journal of Public Health*. 56 (2), 300.

35 Christakis, G. et al. (1966) Effect of the Anti-Coronary Club Program on Coronary Heart Disease Risk-Factor Status. *Journal of American Medical Association*. 198 (6), 597–604.

36 Christakis, G. et al. (1966) Summary of the research activities of the anti-coronary club. *Public Health Reports*. 81 (1), 64–70.

37 Christakis, G. et al. (1966) The anti-coronary club. A dietary approach to the prevention of coronary heart disease–a seven-year report. *American Journal of Public Health*. 56 (2), 299–314.

38 Singman, H. S. et al. (1980) The Anti-Coronary Club : 1957 to 1972. *The American Journal of Clinical Nutrition.* (33), 1183–1191.

39 Teicholz, N. (2014) The Questionable Link Between Saturated Fat and Heart Disease. *Wall Street Journal.* 6 May. [online]. Available from: http://www.wsj.com/articles/SB100014240527 02303678404579533760760481486.

40 Keys, A. (1970) I. The Study Program and Objectives. *Circulation.* 41 (4S1).

41 Kesse, E. et al. (2005) Regional dietary habits of French women born between 1925 and 1950. *European Journal of Nutrition.* 44 (5), 285–292.

42 Tunstall-Pedoe, H. (2008) The French Paradox : Fact or Fiction? *Dialogues in Cardiovascular Medicine.* 13 (3).

43 Kritchevsky, D. (1990) Protein and Atherosclerosis. *Journal of Nutritional Science and Vitaminology.* 36 (5), 81–86.

44 Story, J. A. & Klurfeld, D. M. (2007) David Kritchevsky (1920–2006). *The Journal of Nutrition.* 137 (6), 1355.

45 Story, J. A. & Klurfeld, D. M. (2007) David Kritchevsky (1920–2006). *The Journal of Nutrition.* 137 (6), 1354.

46 Wrangham, R. (2008) *Catching Fire: How Cooking Made Us Human.* Basic Books.

47 Zimmerman, M. R. et al. (1971) Examination of an Aleutian mummy. *Bulletin of the New York Academy of Medicine.* 47 (1), 80.

48 Bishop, K. (2011) Thule palaeopathology: The health concerns of an arctic lifestyle. *Totem: The University of Western Ontario Journal of Anthropology.* 19 (1), 4.

49 Bjerregaarda, P. et al. (2003) Low incidence of cardiovascular disease among the Inuit—what is the evidence? *Atherosclerosis.* 133 (2), 351–357.

50 Zimmerman, M. R. & Aufderheide, A. C. (1984) The Frozen Family of Utqiagvik: The Autopsy Findings. *Artic Anthropology.* 21 (1), 53–64.

51 Teicholz, N. (2014) *The Big Fat Surprise: why butter, meat, and cheese belong in a healthy diet.* Revised Edition. Scribe.

52 Mann, G. V. et al. (1972) Atherosclerosis in the Masai. *American Journal of Epidemiology.* 95 (1), 26.

53 Blackburn, H. (n.d.) *Ancel Keys - by Henry Blackburn, MD* [online]. Available from: http://mbbnet.umn.edu/firsts/blackburn_h.html.

54 Canola Council of Canada (n.d.) *What is Canola? - Canola Council of Canada* [online]. Available from: http://www.canolacouncil.org/oil-and-meal/what-is-canola/ (Accessed 10 December 2016).

55 U.S. Department of Agriculture (1980) *Nutrition and Your Health: Dietary Guidelines for Americans.*

56 Select Committee of Nutrition and Human Needs United States Senate (1977) *Dietary Goals for the United States: Second Edition.*

57 U S Department of Agriculture (2002) *Agriculture Fact Book 2001-2002,* 14-20.

58 U S Department of Agriculture (2002) *Agriculture Fact Book 2001-2002.*

59 Yudkin, J. (1972) *Pure, White and Deadly: the problem of sugar.* London: Davis-Poynter Limited.

60 Truswell, A. S. (2010) *Cholesterol and Beyond: The Research on Diet and Coronary Heart Disease 1900-2000.* Springer Netherlands, 9.2.

61 Truswell, A. S. (2010) *Cholesterol and Beyond: The Research on Diet and Coronary Heart Disease 1900-2000.* Springer Netherlands, 31.4.

62 Keys, A. (1971) Sucrose in the Diet and Coronary Heart Disease. *Atherosclerosis.* 14 (1), 195.

63 Keys, A. (1971) Sucrose in the Diet and Coronary Heart Disease. *Atherosclerosis.* 14 (1), 194.

64 Qing Ye, E. et al. (2012) Greater Whole-Grain Intake is Associated with Lower Risk of Type 2 Diabetes, Cardiovascular Disease, and Weight Gain. *The Journal of Nutrition.* 142 (7), 1304–1313.

65 Steinberg, D. (2007) *The Cholesterol Wars: The Skeptics vs. the Preponderance of Evidence.* San Diego, CA: Academic Press.

66   Country Growers Pty Ltd. (2014) *Extra Virgin Coconut Oil available today!* [online]. Available from: http://countrygrowers. com.au/index.php/blog/44-extra-virgin-coconut-oil-available-today (Accessed 4 August 2016).

67   Cox, C. et al. (1995) Effects of coconut oil, butter, and safflower oil on lipids and lipoproteins in persons with moderately elevated cholesterol levels. *Journal of Lipid Research.* 36 (8), 1787–1795.

68   Reiser, R. et al. (1985) Plasma lipid and lipoprotein response of humans to beef fat, coconut oil and safflower oil1. *American Journal of Clinical Nutrition.* 42 (August), 190–197.

69   Trautwein, E. A. et al. (1997) Effect of dietary fats rich in lauric, myristic, palmitic, oleic or linoleic acid on plasma, hepatic and biliary lipids in cholesterol-fed hamsters. *British Journal of Nutrition.* 77 (4), 605.

70   Blanc, M. et al. (2011) Host defense against viral infection involves interferon mediated down-regulation of sterol biosynthesis. *PLoS Biology.* 9 (3), 1–19.

71   Martin, M. J. et al. (1986) Serum Cholesterol, blood pressure and mortality implications from a cohort of 361 662 men. *The Lancet.* 328 (8513), 933–936.

72   Ballaban-Gil, K. et al. (1998) Complications of the Ketogenic Diet. *Epilepsia.* 39 (7), 744–748.

73   Carroll, K. K. (1975) Experimental Evidence of Dietary Factors and Hormone-dependent Cancers Experimental Evidence of Dietary Factors and Hormone-dependent. *Cancer Research.* 35 (1), 3374–3383.

74   Carroll, K. et al. (1986) Fat and Cancer. *Cancer.* 58 (1), 1818–1825.

75   Tasevska, N. et al. (2012) Sugars in diet and risk of cancer in the NIH-AARP Diet and Health Study. *International Journal of Cancer.* 130 (1), 159–169.

76   Brouwer, I. A. (1991) *Effects of transfatty acid intake on blood lipids and lipoproteins: a systematic review and meta-regression analysis.*

77   Lopez-Garcia, E. et al. (2005) Consumption of Trans Fatty Acids Is Related to Plasma Biomarkers of Inflammation and

Endothelial Dysfunction. American Society for Nutritional Sciences. (October 2004), 562–566.

[78] Ibrahim, A. et al. (2005) Dietary trans-fatty acids alter adipocyte plasma membrane fatty acid composition and insulin sensitivity in rats. *Metabolism.* 54 (2), 240–246.

[79] National Academies of Science (2005) Dietary Reference Intakes for Energy, Carbohydrate, Fiber, Fat, Fatty Acids, Protein and Amino Acids.

[80] Hooper, L. e. et al. (2006) Risks and benefits of omega 3 fats for mortality, cardiovascular disease, and cancer: systematic review. *British Medical Journal.* 332 (7544), 752–760.

[81] Cundiff, D. K. et al. (2007) Relation of Omega-3 Fatty Acid Intake to Other Dietary Factors Known to Reduce Coronary Heart Disease Risk. *American Journal of Cardiology.* 99 (9), 1230–1233.

[82] Dyerberg, J. & Bang, H. O. (1979) Haemostatic function and platelet polyunsaturated fatty acids in Eskimos. Lancet. 2(8140) (Sep 1), 433–435.

[83] Essential amino acids are leucine, isoleucine, valine, lysine, threonine, tryptophan, methionine, phenylalanine and histidine. Non-essential amino acids are alanine, arginine, asparagine, aspartic acid, cysteine, selenocysteine, glutamic acid, glutamine, glycine, proline, serine, and tyrosine.

[84] Campbell, T. C. & Campbell, T. M. (2006) The China Study. Dallas USA: Benbella Books, 27.

[85] Maynard, L. A. (1962) Wilbur O. Atwater (1844-1907). *The Journal of Nutrition,* 78.

[86] Maynard, L. A. (1962) Wilbur O. Atwater (1844-1907). *The Journal of Nutrition,* 78.

[87] Chittenden, R. H. (1904) *Physiological economy in nutrition, with special reference to the minimal protein requirement of the healthy man. An experimental study.* New York: Frederick A. Stokes Company.

[88] National Health and Medical Research Council (2005) Nutrient Reference Values for Australia and New Zealand Including DRI, 29-31.

89   WHO Expert Consultation (2007) Protein and Amino Acid Requirements in Human Nutrition.

90   National Health and Medical Research Council (2005) Nutrient Reference Values for Australia and New Zealand Including DRI. p5, p20 – Reference weight for males with BMI of 22.0 and a moderate activity level requiring energy of 12.0 MJ/day (2900 kcal/day).

91   Sweeney, J. S. (1927) Dietary Factors that Influence the Dextrose Tolerance Test. *Archives of Internal Medicine.* 40 (6), 818–830.

92   Sweeney, J. S. (1928) A comparison of the effects of general diets and of standardized diets on tolerance for dextrose. *Archives of Internal Medicine.* 42 (6), 872–876.

93   Barnard, N. D. et al. (2006) A Low-Fat Vegan Diet Improves Glycemic Control and Cardiovascular Risk Factors in a Randomized Clinical Trial in Individuals With Type 2 Diabetes. *Diabetes Care.* 29 (8), 1777–1783.

94   Memon, R. A. & Gilani, A. H. (1995) An Update on Hyperlipidlemia and its Management. *Journal of Pakistan Medical Association.*

95   Esselstyn, C. B. (2007) Prevent and Reverse Heart Disease. New York: Penguin Group, 30-32.

96   Esselstyn, C. B. (2007) Prevent and Reverse Heart Disease. New York: Penguin Group, 41-43.

97   Vogel, R. A. et al. (1997) Effect of a Single High-Fat Meal on Endothelial Function in Healthy Subjects. *American Journal of Cardiology.* 79 (3), 350–354.

98   Simopoulos, A. P. (1991) Omega-3 fatty acids in health and disease and in growth and development. *The American Journal of Clinical Nutrition.* 54 (3), 438–463.

99   Steinberg, D. (2007) *The Cholesterol Wars: The Skeptics vs. the Preponderance of Evidence.* San Diego, CA: Academic Press.

100 Dobbin, E. V. et al. (1951) The Low-Fat, Low-Cholesterol Diet. Doubleday, Garden City, NY.

101 Tunstall-Pedoe, H. (2008) The French Paradox : Fact or Fiction? *Dialogues in Cardiovascular Medicine.* 13 (3).

102 Kalm, L. M. & Semba, R. D. (2005) They starved so that others be better fed: remembering Ancel Keys and the Minnesota experiment. *The Journal of nutrition*. 135 (6), 1347–1352.

103 Blackburn, H. (n.d.) *Ancel Keys - by Henry Blackburn, MD* [online]. Available from: http://mbbnet.umn.edu/firsts/blackburn_h.html.

104 Keys, A. (1995) Mediterranean diet and public health : personal reflections. *American Journal of Clinical Nutrition*. 613–5.

105 Keys, A. (1953) Atherosclerosis: a problem in newer public health. *Journal of Mt Sinai Hospital*. July-Aug; 20 (2), 122.

106 Keys, A. & Keys, M. (1975) *How to eat well and stay well the Mediterranean way*. Doubleday, Garden City, NY.

107 Williams, R. (2010) Profiles in Cardiovascular Science Joseph Goldstein and Michael Brown Demoting Egos, Promoting Success. *Circulation Research*. 106 (6), 1006–1010.

108 Steinberg, D. (2007) *The Cholesterol Wars: The Skeptics vs. the Preponderance of Evidence*. San Diego, CA: Academic Press.

109 Brown, M. S. et al. (197909-01) Reversible Accumulation Of Cholesteryl Esters In Macrophages Incubated With Acetylated Lipoproteins. *Journal of Cell Biology*. 82 (3), 597–613.

110 National Heart Blood and Lung Institute (2015) *Framingham Heart Study* [online]. Available from: https://www.framinghamheartstudy.org/about-fhs/history.php (Accessed 21 November 2015).

111 National Heart Blood and Lung Institute (2015) *Framingham Heart Study - Intermittent Claudication* [online]. Available from: https://www.framinghamheartstudy.org/risk-functions/intermittent-claudication/index.php (Accessed 21 November 2015).

112 Morrison, L. M. (1955) A Nutritional Program for Prolongation of Life in Coronary Atherosclerosis. *Journal of American Medical Association*. 159 (15), 1425–1428.

113 Morrison, L. M. (1960) Diet in Coronary Atherosclerosis. *Journal of American Medical Association*. 173 (8), 880–884.

114 Yerushalmy, J. & Hilleboe, H. E. (1957) Fat in the Diet and Mortality from Heart Disease. *New York State Journal of Medicine.* 57 (14), 2343–2354.

115 Strom, A. & Jensen, R. A. (1951) Mortality from Circulatory Diseases in Norway 1940-1945. *The Lancet.* 1 (6647), 126–129.

116 Tunstall-Pedoe, H. (2008) The French Paradox : Fact or Fiction? *Dialogues in Cardiovascular Medicine.* 13 (3), 159–179.

117 Kinch, S. H. et al. (1963) Risk factors in ischemic heart disease. *American Journal of Public Health.* 53 (3), 438–442.

118 Jolliffe, N. & Archer, M. (1959) Statistical associations between international coronary heart disease death rates and certain environmental factors. *Journal of Chronic Diseases.* 9 (6).

119 Jolliffe, N. (1959) Fats, Cholesterol, and Coronary Heart Disease. *Circulation.* 20 (1), 109–127.

120 Dayton, S. et al. (196911-16) A Controlled Clinical Trial of a Diet High in Unsaturated Fat in Preventing Complications of Atherosclerosis. *The Lancet.* 292 (7577), 1060–1062.

121 Steinberg, D. (2007) *The Cholesterol Wars: The Skeptics vs. the Preponderance of Evidence.* San Diego, CA: Academic Press.

122 Gillespie, D. (2013) *Toxic Oil: Why Vegetable Oil Will Kill You & How to Save Yourself.* Viking.

123 Karvonen, M. J. (1972) Modification of the diet in primary prevention trials. *The Proceedings of the Nutrition Society.* 31 (1), 355–362.

124 Jolliffe, N. (1959) Fats, Cholesterol, and Coronary Heart Disease. *Circulation.* 20 (1), 109–127.

125 Artaud-Wild, S. M. et al. (1993) Differences in coronary mortality can be explained by differences in cholesterol and saturated fat intakes in 40 countries but not in France and Finland. A paradox. *Circulation.* 88 (6), 2771–2779.

126 Cottel, D. et al. (2000) The North–East–South gradient of coronary heart disease mortality and case fatality rates in France is consistent with a similar gradient in risk factor clusters. *European Journal of Epidemiology.* 16 (4), 317–322.

127 Kesse, E. et al. (2005) Regional dietary habits of French women born between 1925 and 1950. *European Journal of Nutrition*. 44 (5), 285–292.

128 Fromont, A. et al. (2010) Geographic variations of multiple sclerosis in France. *Brain : A Journal of Neurology*. 133 (Pt 7), 1889–1899.

129 Keys, A. et al. (1980) *Seven Countries: A Multivariate Analysis of Death and Coronary Heart Disease*. Cambridge, Massachusetts and London, England: Harvard University Press.

130 Keys, A. et al. (1980) *Seven Countries: A Multivariate Analysis of Death and Coronary Heart Disease*. Cambridge, Massachusetts and London, England: Harvard University Press, 341.

131 Le, L. & Sabate, J. (2014) Beyond Meatless, the Health Effects of Vegan Diets: Findings from the Adventist Cohorts. *Nutrients*. 6 (6), 2131–2147, Table 2.

132 Jacobsen, B. K. et al. (2009) Age at menarche, total mortality and mortality from ischaemic heart disease and stroke: the Adventist Health Study, 1976-88. *International Journal of Epidemiology*. 38 (1), 245–252.

133 Buettner, D. (2012) *The Blue Zones*. Second Ed. Washington DC: National Geographic.

134 Le, L. & Sabate, J. (2014) Beyond Meatless, the Health Effects of Vegan Diets: Findings from the Adventist Cohorts. *Nutrients*. 6 (6), 2131–2147.

135 Kris-Etherton, P. et al. (2001) Lyon Diet Heart Study. *Circulation*. 103 (13), 1823–1825.

136 de Lorgeril, M. et al. (1999) Mediterranean diet, traditional risk factors, and the rate of cardiovascular complications after myocardial infarction: final report of the Lyon Diet Heart Study. *Circulation*. 99 (6), 779–785.

137 Kjelsberg, M. O. et al. (1997) Brief description of the Multiple Risk Factor Intervention Trial. *American Journal of Clinical Nutrition*. 65 (supp), 191S–195S.

138 van Brummelen, P. et al. (1979) Influence of hydrochlorothiazide on the plasma levels of triglycerides, total cholesterol and

HDL-cholesterol in patients with essential hypertension. *Current Medical Research and Opinion.* 6 (1), 24–29.

139 Ernst, M. E. et al. (2011) Long-term effects of chlorthalidone versus hydrochlorothiazide on electrocardiographic left ventricular hypertrophy in the Multiple Risk Factor Intervention Trial. *Hypertension.* 58 (6), 1001–1007.

140 Stamler, J. et al. (2008) The Multiple Risk Factor Intervention Trial (MRFIT)—Importance Then and Now. *Journal of American Medical Association.* 300 (11), 1343–1345.

141 Stamler, J. et al. (2008) The Multiple Risk Factor Intervention Trial (MRFIT)—Importance Then and Now. *Journal of American Medical Association.* 300 (11), 1343–1345.

142 Dolecek, T. A. (1992) Epidemiological Evidence of Relationships between Dietary Polyunsaturated Fatty Acids and Mortality in the Multiple Risk Factor Intervention Trial. *Experimental Biology and Medicine.* 200 (2), 177–182.

143 Women's Health Initiative (n.d.) *Women's Health Initiative* [online]. Available from: https://www.whi.org/about/SitePages/Dietary%20Trial.aspx. (Accessed 3 October 2015).

144 Howard, B. V et al. (2006) Low-Fat Dietary Pattern and Risk of Cardiovascular Disease. *Journal of American Medical Association.* 295 (6), 655–666

145 Puska, P. et al. (2009) Report Number: 9789522450005. *The North Karelia Project: From North Karelia to National Action.* National Institute for Health and Welfare (THL).

146 Blackburn, H. W. (1995) *On the Trail of Heart Attacks in Seven Countries.* Minnesota: University of Minnesota. [online]. Available from: http://sph.umn.edu/site/docs/epi/SPH%20Seven%20Countries%20Study.pdf (Accessed 3 June 2016).

147 Physicians' Health Study (n.d.) *Physicians' Health Study Web Site* [online]. Available from: http://phs.bwh.harvard.edu/index.html.

148 Djoussé, L. & Gaziano, J. M. (2008) Egg consumption in relation to cardiovascular disease and mortality: the Physicians' Health Study. *American Journal of Clinical Nutrition.* 87 (4), 964–969.

[149] Mann, J. I. et al. (1997) Dietary determinants of ischaemic heart disease in health conscious individuals. *Heart.* 78 (5), 450–455.

[150] National Heart Foundation of Australia (n.d.) *Eggs - The Heart Foundation* [online]. Available from: http://heartfoundation. org.au/healthy-eating/food-and-nutrition/protein-foods/eggs (Accessed 18 February 2016).

[151] Karjalainen, J. et al. (1992) A Bovine Albumin Peptide as a possible trigger of insulin-dependent Diabetes Mellitus. *New England Journal of Medicine.* 327 (5), 302–307.

[152] Saukkonen, T. et al. (1994) Children With Newly Diagnosed IDDM Have Increased Levels of Antibodies to Bovine Serum Albumin But Not to Ovalbumin. *Diabetes Care.* 17 (9), 970–976.

[153] Levy-Marchal, C. et al. (1995) Antibodies against bovine albumin and other diabetes markers in French children. *Diabetes Care.* 18 (8), 1089–1094.

[154] Dahl-Jorgensen, K. et al. (1991) Relationship Between Cows' Milk Consumption and Incidence of IDDM in Childhood. *Diabetes Care.* 14 (11), 1081–1083.

[155] Karjalainen, J. et al. (1992) A Bovine Albumin Peptide as a possible trigger of insulin-dependent Diabetes Mellitus. *New England Journal of Medicine.* 327 (5), 302–307.

[156] Campbell, T. C. & Campbell, T. M. (2006) *The China Study.* Dallas USA: Benbella Books.

[157] Doll, R. & Li, L. (1993) *The China Project-Summary Statistics. Full Names and Abbreviations for all 639 Variables,* 19–103.

[158] U.S. Department of Agriculture (2014) *What We Eat in America, NHANES 2011-2012.*

[159] Campbell, T. C. & Campbell, T. M. (2006) *The China Study.* Dallas USA: Benbella Books, 87.

[160] Banting, W. (1864) *Letter on Corpulence.* Third Edit. London: Harrison, 59 Pall Mall.

[161] Evans, F. A. (1947) 'Obesity', in Garfield G. Duncan (ed.) *Diseases of Metabolism: Detailed Methods of Diagnosis and Treatment. A Text for the Practitioner.* Second Edition Philadelphia and London: W. B. Saunders Company.

[162] Taubes, G. (2009) *The Diet Delusion.* London: Vermilion.

¹⁶³ Katovsky, B. (2011) *The Dukan Diet and the History of Dieting* [online]. Available from: http://fyiliving.com/diet/weight-loss/the-dukan-diet-and-the-history-of-dieting/ (Accessed 21 November 2015).

¹⁶⁴ Funding Universe (2004) *History of Atkins Nutritionals Inc* [online]. Available from: http://www.fundinguniverse.com/company-histories/atkins-nutritionals-inc-history/. (Accessed 1 June 2015).

¹⁶⁵ Gordon, E. S. et al. (1963) A New Concept in the Treatment of Obesity. *Journal of American Medical Association*. 186 (1), 50–60.

¹⁶⁶ McLaughlin, K. & Winslow, R. (2004) Report Details Dr. Atkins's Health Problems. *New York Journal*. 10 February. [online]. Available from: http://www.wsj.com/articles/SB107637899384525268. (Accessed 23 November 2015).

¹⁶⁷ Sears, B. (2008) *Toxic fat: when good fat turns bad*. Nashville, Tennessee: Thomas Nelson Inc.

¹⁶⁸ Sears, B. (2013) Don't confuse me with the facts [online]. Available from: http://www.zonediet.com/blog/dont-confuse-me-with-the-facts/ (Accessed 2 June 2015).

¹⁶⁹ Sears, B. (2016) *Dietary Program to Reduce Inflammation* [online]. Available from: http://www.zonediet.com/the-zone-diet/ (Accessed 8 December 2016).

¹⁷⁰ Agaston, A. (2003) *South Beach Diet*. Rodale Press, Inc.

¹⁷¹ Dukan, P. (n.d.) *Dukan Diet* [online]. Available from: www.dukandiet.com/ (Accessed 2 June 2015).

¹⁷² Voegtlin, W. L. (1975) *The Stone Age Diet*. Vantage Press.

¹⁷³ Eaton, S. B. & Konner, M. (1985) Paleolithic Nutrition - A Consideration of its Nature and Current Implications. *New England Journal of Medicine*. (312), 283–289.

¹⁷⁴ Eaton, S. B. et al. (1988) *The Paleolithic Prescription: A Program of Diet & Exercise and a Design for Living*. New York: Harper & Row.

¹⁷⁵ Colorado State University (n.d.) *Loren Cordain - Colorado State University* [online]. Available from: http://www.hes.chhs.colostate.edu/faculty-staff/cordain.aspx (Accessed 21 November 2015).

176 Vandyken, P. (2015) *What to Eat on the Paleo Diet* [online]. Available from: http://thepaleodiet.com/what-to-eat-on-the-paleo-diet-paul-vandyken/ (Accessed 21 November 2015).

177 Cordain, L. (2010) *The Paleo Diet*. Revised. John Wiley & Sons Ltd.

178 Bisht, B. et al. (2014) A multimodal intervention for patients with secondary progressive multiple sclerosis: feasibility and effect on fatigue. *Journal of Alternative and Complementary Medicine* 20 (5), 347–355.

179 Milton, K. (2002) 'Hunter-Gatherer Diets: Wild Foods Signal Relief from Diseases of Affluence', in Peter S. Ungar & Mark F. Teaford (eds.) *Human Diet - Its Origin and Evolution*. 113.

180 Milton, K. (2002) 'Hunter-Gatherer Diets: Wild Foods Signal Relief from Diseases of Affluence', in Peter S. Ungar & Mark F. Teaford (eds.) *Human Diet - Its Origin and Evolution*. 114.

181 Milton, K. (1999) Nutritional Characteristics of Wild Primate Foods: Do the Diets of Our Closest Living Relatives Have Lessons for Us? *Nutrition*.

182 Milton, K. (2003) Micronutrient intakes of wild primates: are humans different? *Comparative Biochemistry and Physiology*. 49.

183 Milton, K. (2000) *Hunter-gatherer diets - a different perspective*. 667.

184 Segurela, L. et al. (2012) The ABO blood group is a trans-species polymorphism in primates. *Proceedings of the National Academy of Sciences*. 109 (45), 18493–18498.

185 Furukawa, T. (1929) A Study of Temperament and Blood-Groups. *Journal of Social Psychology*. 1 (4), 494–509.

186 Wang, J. et al. (2014) ABO Genotype, 'Blood-Type' Diet and Cardiometabolic Risk Factors. *PLoS ONE*. 9 (1), e84749.

187 U.S. Department of Agriculture (2010) *What We Eat in America, NHANES 2009-2010*.

188 Anon (n.d.) The DASH Diet for Healthy Weight Loss, Lower Blood Pressure & Cholesterol [online]. Available from: http://dashdiet.org/default.asp (Accessed 15 October 2016).

189 Sacks, F. M. et al. (1974) Blood Pressure in Vegetarians. *American Journal of Epidemiology*. 100 (5), 390–398.

190   Sacks, F. M. et al. (1975) Plasma Lipids and Lipoproteins in Vegetarians and Controls. *New England Journal of Medicine.* 292 (22), 1148–1151.

191   Sacks, F. M. et al. (1981) Effect of Ingestion of Meat on Plasma Cholesterol of Vegetarians. *Journal of American Medical Association.* 246 (6), 640–646.

192   Sacks, F. & Kass, H. (1988) Low blood pressure in vegetarians: effects of specific foods and nutrients. *American Journal of Clinical Nutrition.* 48 (3), 795–800.

193   Appel, L. J. et al. (1997) A clinical trial of the effects of dietary patterns on blood pressure. *New England Journal of Medicine.* 336 (16), 1117–1124.

194   Karanja, N. et al. (1999) Descriptive Characteristics of the Dietary Patterns Used in the Dietary Approaches to Stop Hypertension Trial. *Journal of the American Dietetic Association.* 99 (8), S19–S27.

195   American Heart Association (2015) *The American Heart Association's Diet and Lifestyle Recommendations* [online]. Available from: http://www.heart.org/HEARTORG/HealthyLiving/HealthyEating/Nutrition/The-American-Heart-Associations-Diet-and-Lifestyle-Recommendations_UCM_305855_Article.jsp#.WBFu-i194wc (Accessed 27 October 2016).

196   U.S. Department of Agriculture (2014) *What We Eat in America, NHANES 2011-2012.* [online]. Available from: https://www.ars.usda.gov/nea/bhnrc/fsrg. Table 1 Calculated from data used for males and females aged 30-39.

197   Swain, J. F. et al. (2008) Characteristics of the Diet Patterns Tested in the Optimal Macronutrient Intake Trial to Prevent Heart Disease (OmniHeart): Options for a Heart-Healthy Diet. *Journal of the Academy of Nutrition and Dietetics.* 108 (2), 257–265.

198   McDougall, J. et al. (2014) Effects of 7 days on an ad libitum low-fat vegan diet: the McDougall Program cohort. *Nutrition Journal.* 13 (99), 1–7.

199 Keys, A. (1995) Mediterranean diet and public health : personal reflections. *American Journal of Clinical Nutrition.* 61 (6), 1321S–1323S.

200 Trichopoulou, A. & Vasilopoulou, E. (2000) Mediterranean diet and longevity. *British Journal of Nutrition.* 84 (6), 205–209.

201 Trichopoulou, A. et al. (2009) Anatomy of health effects of Mediterranean diet: Greek EPIC prospective cohort study. *British Medical Journal.* 338 (1), b2337.

202 Buettner, D. (2012) *The Blue Zones.* Second Ed. Washington DC: National Geographic.

203 Carr, D. (1847) Kessinger Publishing, LLC. *The necessity of brown bread for digestion, nourishment, and sound health, and the injurious effects of white bread.* London: Effingham Wilson.

204 McDougall, J. (2013) *Nathan Pritikin - McDougall's Most Important Mentor* [online]. Available from: https://www. drmcdougall.com/misc/2013nl/feb/pritikin.htm (Accessed 3 June 2015).

205 Anderson, J. et al. (1987) Dietary fiber and diabetes: a comprehensive review and practical application. *Journal of the American Dietetic Association.* 87 (9).

206 Roberts, W. C. (1991) We think we are one, we act as if we are one, but we are not one. *American Journal of Cardiology.* 66 (10), 896.

207 Roberts, W. C. (2010) It's the cholesterol, stupid! *American Journal of Cardiology.* 106 (9), 57.

208 ABC - Audience and Consumer Affairs (2014) *Catalyst Heart of the Matter Investigation Report,* 1–49.

209 Yerushalmy, J. & Hilleboe, H. E. (1957) Fat in the Diet and Mortality from Heart Disease. *New York State Journal of Medicine.* 57 (14), 2343–2354.

210 Keys, A. (1995) Mediterranean diet and public health : personal reflections. *American Journal of Clinical Nutrition.* 61 (6), 1321S–1323S.

211 Keys, A. (1953) Atherosclerosis: a problem in newer public health. *Journal of Mt Sinai Hospital.* July-Aug; 20 (2), 118–139.

[212] Steinberg, D. (2007) *The Cholesterol Wars: The Skeptics vs. the Preponderance of Evidence.* San Diego, CA: Academic Press.

[213] Truswell, A. S. (2010) *Cholesterol and Beyond: The Research on Diet and Coronary Heart Disease 1900-2000.* Springer Netherlands.

[214] Truswell, A. S. (2003) *ABC of Nutrition.* Fourth Edition. London: BMJ Publishing Group.

[215] Mann, J. & Truswell, A. S. (eds.) (2012) *Essentials of Human Nutrition.* Fourth Edition. London: Oxford University Press.

[216] Dixon, J. L. (2015) *Genius and Partnership Ancel and Margaret Keys and the Discovery of The Mediterranean Diet.* New Brunswick, NJ: Joseph L. Dixon Publishing.

Index